Word Eaters: Graphophagy in the Early and High Middle Ages

Mini-Monographs in Medieval and Early Modern Studies

VOLUME 6

The titles published in this series are listed at *brill.com/mini*

Word Eaters

Graphophagy in the Early and High Middle Ages

By

Andrea Maraschi

BRILL

ISSN 2949-8686
ISBN 978-90-04-76549-8
ISBN 978-90-04-76552-8 (PDF)
DOI https://doi.org/10.1163/9789004765528

Library of Congress Control Number: 2026940840

Brill and Koninklijke Brill BV are part of De Gruyter Brill.
www.degruyterbrill.com

Questions about General Product Safety Regulation: productsafety@degruyterbrill.com

Cover illustration: Ezekiel eats the bittersweet scroll containing a prophecy for the Israelites (illuminated initial E). Paris, BNF, MS Latin 16744, fol. 81r. Source: gallica.bnf.fr – Bibliothèque nationale de France.

Contents

Figures

Introduction: Hungry for Words

This book investigates a practice that was widespread yet rarely conceptualised as such in medieval Europe: the ingestion of written and spoken words for therapeutic, protective, divinatory, or transformative purposes. I refer to this practice as *graphophagy*, a term coined here from the Greek *graphein* (γράφειν, "to write") and *phagein* (φαγεῖν, "to eat"), to denote the ritualised consumption of letters, words, or formulae.[1] Related terms such as *logophagy* ("ingestion of words") or *bibliophagy* ("ingestion of books") exist in other scholarly traditions, yet none has been systematically applied to medieval Europe or employed as an analytical category capable of bringing together dispersed and marginal evidence.[2] By introducing graphophagy as a heuristic concept, this study seeks to identify, contextualise, and interpret a set of practices that have so far remained largely invisible within medieval studies.

The ingestion of words may appear alien from a modern perspective, yet medieval sources attest to its persistence from late antiquity through the high and later Middle Ages. In the early Middle Ages, recipes for healing, divination, protection, and love circulated among both the literate and the illiterate, with clerics frequently involved in their transmission and use. These practices did not necessarily entail a rejection of Christianity; on the contrary, Christian words, objects, and ritual frameworks were often fully integrated into them.[3] Graphophagic practices, in particular, surface in sources that are rarely examined together – medical recipes, collections of charms, theological polemic, hagiographic and saga literature, early legal texts, and more. They are found across different linguistic, cultural, and confessional contexts, and were employed by clerics and laypeople, healers and physicians alike. Although graphophagic practices were widespread, they were probably perceived as an alternative or emergency measure. They had no clear precedent within Judeo-Christian tradition, and the few instances of word ingestion that do appear there were either allegorical or residual survivals of earlier cultural practices, as will be shown.

1 Giorgio R. Cardona, "Gli amuleti scritti: un excursus comparativo," *La Ricerca Folklorica* 8 (1983): 91–97; Giorgio R. Cardona, *Antropologia della scrittura* (Utet, 2009 [1981]), 145.

2 On the distinct practice of bibliotherapy, see instead: Paul Gerhard Schmidt, "Il libro come medicina: la biblioterapia," trans. Iolanda Ventura, in *Terapie e guarigioni. Convegno internazionale (Ariano Irpino, 5–7 Ottobre 2008)*, ed. Agostino Paravicini Bagliani (SISMEL – Edizioni del Galluzzo, 2010), 55–63.

3 Bernadette Filotas, *Pagan Survivals: Superstitions and Popular Cultures in Early Medieval Pastoral Literature* (Pontifical Institute of Mediaeval Studies, 2005), 15–16.

 | HTTPS://DOI.ORG/10.1163/9789004765528-002

The primary aim of this book is to reconstruct the circulation and uses of graphophagic practices in the early and high medieval West, roughly from late antiquity to the twelfth century, while occasionally referring to earlier and later chronologies for nuance. The book is meant to demonstrate that the ingestion of textual matter was neither culturally isolated nor conceptually incoherent, but rather part of a broader Mediterranean and European history of embodied textual practices. Given the fragmentary and uneven nature of the evidence, this study does not claim to offer an exhaustive catalogue of graphophagic remedies. Instead, it seeks to identify recurring patterns, shared assumptions, and culturally meaningful variations. Why should the practice of ingesting words be significant to medieval historians, though?

First, graphophagy was *unusual* – not impractical, but distinctively *other*. Second, it was remarkably *adaptable*. Belief in the efficacy of words, across languages, allowed ancient terms and formulae referencing older deities to persist, concentrating extralinguistic forces onto edible surfaces or philtres. Finally, graphophagy reflects *universal* cognitive processes[4] – analogical reasoning and belief in supernatural agency appear common to all human groups, suggesting they may have evolved as adaptive traits.[5] Word ingestion naturally followed from this proclivity.

Now, not only has there been a lack of specific studies on graphophagy,[6] but it is also relevant to those interested in the history of magic, science, and religion, as well as to those engaged in innovative perspectives on food history. This has been shown, for instance, in a recent workshop organized jointly by the University of Fribourg and New York University on May 23–24, 2024 (and, specifically, by Jérémie Koering and Finbarr Barry Flood).

The most challenging aspect of researching graphophagy is the nature of its focus, since graphophagic remedies belong to that subset of practices based on verbal or written formulae believed to possess protective, curative, or apotropaic power, loosely addressed as "charms." Several examples will concern

4 Leonard Zusne and Warren H. Jones, *Anomalistic Psychology: A Study of Magical Thinking* (L. Erlbaum, 1989); Jesper Sørensen, *A Cognitive Theory of Magic* (Altamira Press, 2007), 2; Karl S. Rosengren and Jason A. French, "Magical Thinking," in *The Oxford Handbook of the Development of Imagination*, ed. Marjorie Taylor (Oxford University Press, 2013), 42–60.

5 Phillips Stevens Jr., *Rethinking the Anthropology of Magic and Witchcraft. Inherently Human* (Routledge, 2024), 2. On the problem of unalleviated fears see Susan Mineka and Arne Öhman, "Phobias and Preparedness: The Selective, Automatic, and Encapsulated Nature of Fear," *Biological Psychiatry* 52, no. 10 (2002): 927–37.

6 See, for instance, Michael D. Swartz, "Magical Piety in Ancient and Medieval Judaism," in *Ancient Magic and Ritual Power*, ed. Marvin Meyer and Paul Mirecki (Brill, 2001), 167–84, at 178; David Frankfurter, "The Theory and Practice of the Magical *Historiola* in Ritual Spells," in ibid., 455–76, at 467.

a subcategory of these: medical charms.[7] However, the goal of this study is to analyse cases of ingestion of any type of words and formulae, which require transcending the conceptual boundaries of "charm" as currently defined in scholarship. Remedies in our manuscripts recommend ingesting several textual typologies which were attributed a specific *virtus*.[8]

Locating edible formulae is challenging. They appear scattered across manuscripts of varied content – sometimes deliberately concealed, often as marginal or isolated cases. Their meaning and context are difficult to interpret, and tracing their evolution is problematic given uneven attestations across Western Europe and the practice's appearance in diverse religious and practical contexts.

Enigmatic letters and words – whether spoken or written – continued to be consumed between late antiquity and the late Middle Ages.[9] They were often regarded as functional, intended to "change" the world or act upon it and alter reality by empowering food and drink.[10] In many circumstances, cures relied solely on characters, names, and formulae, suggesting that their origins lay in a synthesis of learned and popular practices. While the use of written texts was associated with elite practitioners and monastic centres, the logic underlying graphophagy appears closely related to "the folk tradition of oral performance."[11]

Recent scholarship on charms, particularly regarding Anglo-Saxon England, has adopted similar approaches. Given textual ingestion's peripheral nature, though, I have pursued a comparative perspective across a substantial manuscript corpus. The bibliography includes only those containing clear traces of graphophagy. By no means do I claim to offer a comprehensive analysis of the phenomenon under examination. I nonetheless hope this study will shed

7 Carrie Griffin, "Historiography of Medieval Medicine," in *Handbook of Medieval Studies*, 651–66, at 656. On this, see also J.H.G. Grattan and Charles Singer, *Anglo-Saxon Magic and Medicine* (Oxford University Press, 1952).

8 On charms in medicinal recipe collections, see Edina Bozóky, "Medieval Narrative Charms," in *The power of Words. Studies on Charms and Charming in Europe*, ed. James Kapaló, Éva Pócs, and William Ryan (Central European University Press, 2013), 101–15, at 105–6.

9 Cf. Russell Poole, "Charms and Incantations," in *Handbook of Medieval Studies*, 1700–1705, at 1704.

10 Leslie K. Arnovick, *Verbal Medicines. The Curative Power of Prayer and Invocation in Early English Charms* (Cambridge University Press, 2024), 239; Audrey L. Meaney, "Extra-medical Elements in Anglo-Saxon Medicine," *Social History of Medicine* 24, no. 1 (2011): 41–56, at 42.

11 Arnovick, *Verbal Medicines*, 241.

light on a phenomenon that has so far received very little attention in medieval studies.

Before turning to specific evidence, it is necessary to address a preliminary question: was graphophagy understood by medieval actors as a form of magic?

The question of how to conceptualise practices like graphophagy requires careful attention to the category of "magic" itself – a term with a complex genealogy[12] and whose analytical utility has been vigorously contested.[13] Valerie Flint argued that practices officially condemned as "magic" were progressively Christianised rather than suppressed, suggesting a model of absorption and transformation.[14] However, this framework has drawn criticism for implying that magic existed as a stable phenomenon outside Christianity, waiting to be incorporated.[15] As Yitzhak Hen observes, such practices "were always there, as a social practice, from the beginning of civilisation" and were in fact "part of society's cultural and social heritage" rather than external to it.[16]

This debate matters for graphophagy because it shapes how we may interpret the sources. Adopting Hen's perspective, word ingestion operated within Christian cultural frameworks – however ambiguously positioned – from the outset and required no specific Church strategy for co-option.

Anthropological critique deepens this issue.[17] Stanley Tambiah argued that magic is best understood not as a bounded domain but as a mode of action, while historian of religion Naomi Janowitz has further discouraged the use of

---

12 Naomi Janowitz, *Magic in the Roman World. Pagans, Jews and Christians* (Routledge, 2001), 9–10.

13 Joseph Bidez and Franz Cumont, *Les mages hellénisés* (Les Belles Lettres, 1939); Elias J. Bickerman, "Darius I, Pseudo-Smerdis, and the Magi," *Athenaeum* 58 (1978): 239–61; Marvin Meyer and Paul Mirecki, "Introduction," in *Ancient Magic and Ritual Power*, 1–11, at 2; Marvin Meyer and Richard Smith, "Introduction," in *Ancient Christian Magic. Coptic Texts of Ritual Power*, ed. Marvin Meyer and Richard Smith (HarperCollins, 1994), 1–9, at 2; Owen Davies, *Magic: A Very Short Introduction* (Oxford University Press, 2012), 41; Peter Brown, *Religion and Society in the Age of Saint Augustine* (Faber&Faber, 1972), 126.

14 Valerie I.J. Flint, *The Rise of Magic in Early Medieval Europe* (Princeton University Press, 1991).

15 Bengt Ankarloo and Stuart Clark, "Introduction," in *Witchcraft and Magic in Europe: 3. The Middle Ages*, ed. Karen L. Jolly, Catharina Raudvere, and Edward Peters (The Athlone Press, 2002), ix–xiv. See also Rob Meens, "Magic and the Early Medieval World View," in *The Community, the Family, and the Saint. Patterns of Power in Early Medieval Europe*, ed. Joyce M. Hill and Mary Swan (Brepols, 1998), 285–95; Richard Kieckhefer, "The Specific Rationality of Medieval Magic," *The American Historical Review* 99, no. 3 (1994): 813–36.

16 Yitzhak Hen, *Culture and Religion in Merovingian Gaul, A.D. 481–751* (Brill, 1995), 159, fn. 26.

17 For a synthesis, see Susan Greenwood, *The Anthropology of Magic* (Berg, 2009), 5; Robert J. Wallis, "Witchcraft and Magic in the Age of Anthropology," in *The Oxford Illustrated History of Witchcraft and Magic*, ed. Owen Davies (Oxford University Press, 2017), 225–52.

essentialist categories.[18] We should instead ask how graphophagy *functioned* within specific contexts.

The sources suggest graphophagic remedies functioned as integrated practice – present in different contexts without apparent anxiety. Yet medieval actors themselves sometimes invoked *magia* and *superstitio* to police boundaries,[19] requiring us to recognise these categories' constructed nature while attending to their historical work. From the twelfth century, moreover, natural magic emerged as a distinct conception grounded in nature's occult properties and celestial influences.[20] Yet condemnatory discourses persisted,[21] and self-referential positive notions of magic from Plotinus and the *Greek Magical Papyri* complicated the picture. This coexistence emphasises *magic*'s instability as a historical category.

From this perspective, practices traditionally labelled as *magical* may be more productively analysed as forms of ritual action. Tambiah's insight that ritual language functions performatively rather than propositionally helps explain why graphophagic formulae need not be understood to be effective.[22] Their logic is frequently analogical and their effectiveness persuasive rather than empirical, yet they constitute internally coherent systems of practice within their cultural contexts.

This concept seems well suited to describe how graphophagy may have been perceived by those who practiced it. The ingestion of words relied on analogical reasoning enabling the transfer of virtues from written signs to bodies. However, in early medieval Europe, ritual and practical efficacy were not always differentiated.[23] Anglo-Saxon remedies – Gospel passages written, dissolved in water, combined with herbs and wine, blessed through multiple masses – operated through multiple registers simultaneously: healing,

18 Stanley J. Tambiah, *Magic, Science, Religion, and the Scope of Rationality* (Cambridge University Press, 1991); Naomi Janowitz, *Icons of Power: Ritual Practices in Late Antiquity* (The Pennsylvania State University Press, 2002), xiii–xiv.

19 Martha Rampton, *Trafficking with Demons. Magic, Ritual, and Gender from Late Antiquity to 1000* (Cornell University Press, 2021), 1–14.

20 Richard Kieckhefer, *Magic in the Middle Ages* (Cambridge University Press, 1989). See also Filotas, *Pagan Survivals*, 285–87.

21 Jeffrey B. Russell, *Witchcraft in the Middle Ages* (Cornell University Press, 1972), 20–3.

22 Stanley J. Tambiah, "Form and meaning of magical acts. A point of view," *Hau: Journal of Ethnographic Theory* 7, no. 3 (2017): 451–73 (orig. pub. in *Modes of thought: Essays on thinking in Western and non-Western societies*, ed. Robin Horton and Ruth Finnegan [London: Faber & Faber, 1973], 199–229).

23 Stanley J. Tambiah, "The Magical Power of Words," *Man* 3, no. 2 (1968): 175–208, 198–202; Id., "A Performative Approach to Ritual," *Proceedings of the British Academy* 65 (1979): 113–69, 129–30.

devotion, penance, and public faith. Words functioned not as simple medical ingredients but as vectors of divine power, textual authority, and bodily transformation.

Word ingestion was never arbitrary but followed formalised rules of timing, inscription, repetition, and execution. Whether performed by clerics, healers, or laypeople, graphophagic acts relied on shared expectations of efficacy and authority.[24] Sources often do not clarify whether practitioners understood efficacy as medical, devotional, or thaumaturgic[25] – reflecting a cultural landscape where such distinctions were fluid. Graphophagy maintained social cohesion by consolidating collective beliefs,[26] ritualised – following Catherine Bell's analysis – through deliberate performance that endowed textual consumption with special efficacy.[27] Though grounded in eating, consumption of words transformed an ordinary biological act into ritualised activity[28] – ritual even without formal institutionalisation.

Sources rarely frame graphophagy as a distinct form of *magic*. Rather, these practices appear fully integrated within broader contexts – as rituals invoking divine entities, techniques for activating the occult or natural properties of substances, therapeutic remedies, or channels of thaumaturgic power. As suggested by Lucy Grig, "rituals allow for the intersection of the sacred and the profane through practice." In this sense, while reflecting religious landscapes, rituals also contributed to their perpetual transformation.[29] This flexibility suggests that graphophagy was not perceived as anomalous, but as a legitimate mode of acting upon the world within established frameworks of meaning.

For all these reasons, in this book I adopt an explicitly contextual and emic approach, privileging neutral descriptive terms (ritual, divinatory, or therapeutic practices) while retaining *magic* only where sources themselves employ it polemically or self-referentially, or where later developments gave it distinct

---

24 Clifford Geertz, *The Interpretation of Cultures: Selected Essays by Clifford Geertz* (Basic Books, 2000 [1973]), 87–125; David I. Kertzer, *Ritual, Politics, and Power* (Yale University Press, 1988), 8ff.

25 Katherine Storm Hindley, *Textual Magic. Charms and Written Amulets in Medieval England* (The University of Chicago Press, 2023), 3–4.

26 Émile Durkheim, *The Elementary Forms of Religious Life*, trans. J.W. Swain (Free Press, 1965 [1915]), 463ff.; Roy A. Rappaport, *Ritual and Religion in the Making of Humanity* (Cambridge University Press, 1999), 23–7.

27 Catherine Bell, *Ritual Theory, Ritual Practice* (Oxford University Press, 2009 [1992]), 7–8.

28 Ibid., 219–20.

29 Lucy Grig, "Life and Death in Late Antiquity: Religious Rituals and Popular Culture," in *A Companion to Religion in Late Antiquity*, ed. Josef Lössl and Nicholas J. Baker-Brian (Wiley Blackwell, 2018), 455–73, at 456.

meanings (e.g., natural magic).[30] This methodological choice reflects not indifference to theoretical debates but recognition that graphophagy's significance lies precisely in its resistance to categorical stability.[31] Rather than treating graphophagy as a subcategory of magic defined *ex ante*, it examines how practices of textual ingestion functioned within their specific textual, ritual, and social environments.

A book on graphophagy must address the assumption – shared by its practitioners – that language possesses extralinguistic power. Writing has long been treated primarily as a technical invention, analysed in terms of its origins, dissemination, and the evolution of graphic systems. However, scholars have shown that writing is one of the privileged domains of ideological and symbolic production within societies. Its cultural significance extends well beyond its instrumental function. Every writing system presents various aspects – cognitive, social, religious, and, in many contexts, what has been described as magical – whose observation allows for a deep understanding of the society that produced them and within which they circulated.[32]

Jack Goody observed that writing instruments become invested with supernatural powers, particularly in religious contexts, encapsulating communicative power for internalisation.[33] Similar principles can be observed throughout late antiquity and the early Middle Ages, in both the Eastern and Western side of the Mediterranean sea, as will be shown. A more specific focus on the powers attributed to words among oral societies characterises the work of Walter Ong, who argued that oral cultures tend to regard words as inherently potent

30 On this approach, see: David L. D'Avray, "The Concept of Magic," in *The Routledge History of Medieval Magic*, ed. Sophie Page and Catherine Rider (Routledge, 2019), 48–56; David Frankfurter, "Ancient Magic in a New Key: Refining an Exotic Discipline in the History of Religions," in *Guide to the Study of Ancient Magic*, ed. David Frankfurter (Brill, 2019), 3–20; Bernd-Christian Otto, "A Discourse Historical Approach Towards Medieval Learned Magic," in *The Routledge History of Medieval Magic*, 37–47. See also Russel T. McCutcheon, *The insider/outsider problem in the Study of Religion* (Cassel, 1999).

31 Jan N. Bremmer, "The Birth of the Term 'Magic,'" *Zeitschrift für Papyrologie und Epigraphik* 126 (1999): 1–12.

32 See: Charles Kay Ogden and Ivor A. Richards. *The Meaning of Meaning* (Kegan Paul, 1923); Bronisław Malinowski, *Coral Gardens and Their Magic*, 2 vols. (Indiana University Press, 1935); Claude Lévi-Strauss, "The Effectiveness of Symbols," in *Structural Anthropology 1*, ed. Claude Lévi-Strauss (Penguin, 1949), 186–205; Maurice Bloch, "Symbols, Song, Dance, and Features of Articulation: Is Religion an Extreme Form of Authority?," *Archives Européennes de Sociologie* 15 (1974): 55–81.

33 Jack Goody, ed., *Literacy in traditional societies* (Cambridge University Press, 1968); Id., "Restricted Literacy in Northern Ghana," in *Literacy in traditional societies*, 198–264, at 230. See also Harry Walker, "On Logophagy and Truth: Interpretation through Incorporation among Peruvian Urarina," *Language & Communication* 63 (2018): 15–22.

precisely because they are sounded and embodied.[34] This potency could be theorised, within certain learned traditions that circulated in medieval Europe alongside the theory of rays attributed to al-Kindī, as a form of physical force.[35] At a less erudite level, where such cosmological explanations were absent, spoken and written formulae nonetheless retained a kind of power capable of solving practical problems.

Yet Goody and Ong approach the question from opposite directions, and the tension between their perspectives sheds light on graphophagy's distinctive character. For Goody, writing's power stems from its material permanence and institutional authority – its capacity to fix knowledge in durable, transportable form. For Ong, power inheres in speech's immediacy and physicality – its embeddedness in the living body.[36] Graphophagy occupies precisely the space where these two forms of power converge: writing made edible becomes simultaneously material and incorporated, permanent inscription rendered biologically temporary through digestion. The practice thus cannot be understood through either framework alone; it requires recognising how medieval cultures maintained both orientations toward language simultaneously.

David Frankfurter has demonstrated that in late antique ritual contexts, writing operated not merely to convey meaning but to materialise power. Letters and words functioned as substances endowed with authority and power – a tendency that was further reinforced by the rise of religions founded on the written word.[37] This framework helps explain graphophagic recipes that specify destruction as the locus of efficacy: texts are written not to endure but to be dissolved, licked away, or swallowed. Yet, Frankfurter's focus on late antiquity leaves open whether similar logics operated in early medieval Europe, where Christianity's emphasis on the incarnate Word created its own theological rationale for materialised textuality.

Beatrice Delaurenti has shown that medieval learned debates about the power of words turned precisely on the questions of materiality and

34 Walter J. Ong, *Orality and Literacy: The Technologizing of the Word* (Methuen, 1982), 31–2. See also Walter J. Ong, *Interfaces of the Word* (Cornell University Press, 1977).

35 Charles Burnett, "The Theory and Practice of Powerful Words in Medieval Magical Texts," in *The Word in Medieval Logic, Theology and Psychology: Acts of the XIII International Colloquium of the Société Internationale pour l'Étude de la Philosophie Médiévale*, Kyoto, 27 September–1 October 2005, ed. Tetsuro Shimizu and Charles Burnett (Brepols, 2009), 215–31.

36 Ong, *Orality and Literacy*, 65–6.

37 David Frankfurter, "The Magic of Writing in Mediterranean Antiquity," in *Guide to the Study of Ancient Magic*, ed. David Frankfurter (Brill, 2019), 626–58, at 626–27.

transmission.[38] Could words act physically, or only symbolically? Did their power derive from inherent properties or divine authorisation? Early medieval authorities repeatedly expressed concern about excessive reliance on words, which they feared might open the gates to demonic influence and expose both practitioners and patients to spiritual danger.[39] Graphophagy sits at the center of these debates: as a practice requiring both material inscription and bodily incorporation, it made unavoidable the question of how words were thought to act.

Despite sustained interest in the powers attributed to writing, the only monograph entirely dedicated to this topic remains Giorgio Cardona's anthropological study.[40] Medievalists, meanwhile, have produced a substantial work on textual or talismanic magic, but graphophagy's distinctive features have remained obscure.[41] The comprehensive studies of textual amulets by Don

38 Beatrice Delaurenti, "Acting through Words in the Middle Ages: Communication and Action in the Debates on the Power of Incantations," *Archives de sciences sociales des religions* 158, no. 2 (2012): 53–71, at 53; Ead., *La Puissance des mots : "Virtus verborum." Débats doctrinaux sur le pouvoir des incantations au Moyen Âge* (Les Éditions du Cerf, 2007).

39 Hindley, *Textual Magic*, 36–7.

40 Cardona, *Antropologia della scrittura*. See also David Frankfurter, "The Magic of Writing and the Writing of Magic. The Power of the Word in Egyptian and Greek Tradition," *Helios* 21 (1994): 189–221. Studies on specific contexts are: Travis Zadeh, "Touching and Ingesting: Early Debates over the Material Qur'an," *Journal of the American Oriental Society* 129, no. 3 (2009): 446–66; Finbarr Barry Flood, "Bodies and Becoming. Mimesis, Mediation, and the Ingestion of the Sacred in Christianity and Islam," in *Sensational Religion. Sensory Cultures in Material Practice*, ed. Sally M. Promey (Yale University Press, 2014), 459–93; Melissa Pritchard, "On Bibliomancy, Anthropodermic Bibliopegy, and The Eating Papers; or, Proust's Porridge," *Speaking Volumes* 63 (2014): 26–35; Alexandros Tsakos, "Materiality and Physicality of Medieval Manuscripts from Christian Nubia," *Cahiers d'études africaines* 236 (2019): 967–92; Andrea Maraschi, Similia similibus curantur. *Cannibalismo, grafofagia e "magia" simpatetica nel Medioevo (500–1500)* (CISAM, 2020); Id., "Sympathetic Graphophagy in Late Medieval Scandinavian Leechbooks and Collections of Charms," in *Civilizations of the Supernatural: Witchcraft, Ritual, and Religious Experience in Late Antique, Medieval, and Renaissance Traditions*, ed. Fabrizio Conti (Trivent Publishing, 2020), 247–64; Id., "Mangiare preghiere, bere incantesimi. Casi di grafofagia religiosa e magica nell'alto Medioevo," in *Medioevo misterioso*, ed. Paola Galetti (Edizioni Scritture, 2024) 99–115; Safet HadžiMuhamedović, "My Grandmother Drank the Qur'an: Liquid Readings and Permeable Bodies in Bosnia," *CounterText* 7, no. 1 (2021): 73–89. On iconophagy, see instead Jérémie Koering, *Les iconophages: Une histoire de l'ingestion des images* (Actes Sud Éditions, 2021); trans. Nicholas Huckle as *Iconophages. A History of Ingesting Images* (Zone Books, 2024).

41 E.g.: Richard Kieckhefer, *Forbidden Rites: A Necromancer's Manual of the Fifteenth Century* (Pennsylvania State University Press, 1998); Claire Fanger, ed., *Conjuring Spirits: Texts and Traditions of Medieval Ritual Magic* (Pennsylvania State University Press, 1998); Roy D.

Skemer examine worn texts rather than consumed ones. He demonstrates that medieval amulets involved complex relationships between text, material support, and bodily proximity, yet he treats ingestion as marginal to his analysis – understandably, since his focus is texts worn on the body.[42] In turn, Edina Bozóky has shown that charms were written down in order to preserve them, to disseminate them, and to be used in written form as individual remedies.[43]

This study builds upon, but also moves beyond, these frameworks. While Goody and Ong emphasise the symbolic authority of writing and speech, and medievalists have examined the inscription and transmission of charms, graphophagy has remained largely untheorised. By focusing on ingestion rather than inscription alone, this book brings these approaches into dialogue and shows how textual efficacy was not only read, heard, or worn, but physically absorbed – a mode that demanded its own ritual logic and raised its own theological problems. This model treats writing as conservative – a technology for fixing oral traditions in stable form. Yet graphophagic practices complicate this framework because they require writing's destruction rather than preservation.

The notion that words "do things" has become familiar through John Austin's theory of performative utterances and its subsequent applications to historical contexts.[44] Yet Austin's framework, developed for modern linguistic contexts, requires careful adaptation to medieval materials. Austin distinguished performatives (utterances that accomplish actions) from constatives (utterances that describe states of affairs). However, graphophagic formulae work precisely by blurring the line between saying and doing, description and enactment.

Naomi Janowitz has shown for Late Antiquity that ritual language was understood as structurally connected to the cosmos – not metaphorically but through real linkages between properly formed speech, divine names, and material effects.[45] For words to act upon the social world, however, their efficacy depended on the recognition of authority: the speaker, performer, or

Kotansky, "Textual Amulets and Writing Traditions in the Ancient World," in *Guide to the Study of Ancient Magic*, ed. David Frankfurter (Brill, 2019), 507–54.

42 Don C. Skemer, *Binding Words. Textual Amulets in the Middle Ages* (The Pennsylvania State University Press, 2006); Id., "Magic Writ: Textual Amulets Worn on the Body for Protection," in *Schriftträger – Textträger: Zur materialen Präsenz des Geschriebenen in frühen Gesellschaften*, ed. Annette Kehnel and Diamantis Panagiotopoulos (De Gruyter, 2015), 127–50.

43 Edina Bozóky, *Charmes et prières apotropaïques* (Brepols, 2003), 67ff.

44 John L. Austin, *How to Do Things With Words* (Harvard University Press, 1962), esp. 12–24.

45 Janowitz, *Icons of Power*, 60–1.

writer had to be acknowledged as entitled to endow words with operative force. Graphophagic practices appear to assume something closer to Janowitz's cosmic performativity: words act not merely because authorities authorise them but because language itself participates in the structure of reality – a view with roots in both Platonic theories of names and Christian theology of the creative Word.

Yet Pierre Bourdieu has shown that even performative efficacy depends on social recognition: a judge's sentence works because institutions back it; a priest's blessing functions because communities acknowledge priestly authority. This means we cannot treat graphophagic formulae as automatically efficacious but must ask who was recognised as authorised to deploy them.[46] The sources suggest shifting configurations of authority: sometimes clerics (whose literacy and ordination granted access to textual power), sometimes healers (whose specialised knowledge commanded trust), sometimes simply tradition itself (formulae that worked because they had "always" worked). Graphophagy thus operated within multiple authority systems simultaneously.

This multi-layered authority helps explain why graphophagic practices could circulate across the boundaries that modern scholarship imposes between "popular" and "learned," "magical" and "medical," "Christian" and "pagan."

The attribution of extra-linguistic power to speech and text – without necessarily framing it as magical – is particularly evident in cultural contexts with strong vernacular traditions, such as medieval Ireland or Iceland.[47] In graphophagy, however, textual power is activated in a distinctive way: through destruction and consumption. This paradox – that writing must be destroyed to work – distinguishes graphophagy from both textual amulets (which function through proximity and visibility) and spoken charms (which act through vocalisation). Katherine Storm Hindley has recently argued that destruction constitutes its own mode of textual efficacy in medieval English charm tradition, and my evidence confirms her insight while extending it geographically and chronologically.[48] The power to destroy writing and thereby activate

46 Pierre Bourdieu, *Ce que parler veut dire: l'économie des échanges linguistiques* (Fayard, 1982), 105.

47 Nicolas Meylan, "The Magical Power of Poetry," *Saga-Book* XXXVII (2013): 43–60. On possible relationships between medieval Ireland and Iceland, see Michael Richter, "Medieval Ireland and Iceland – Worlds Apart?," in *Saluting Aron Gurevich. Essays in History, Literature and Other Related Subjects*, ed. Yelena Mazour-Matusevich and Alexandra Korros (Brill, 2010), 155–66.

48 Katherine Storm Hindley, "Eating Words and Burning Them: The Power of Destruction in Medieval English Charm Texts," in *Zerstörung von Geschriebenem. Historische und*

it appears as a transregional phenomenon, suggesting shared assumptions about how materialised language could be manipulated, incorporated, and made operative through consumption. Sometimes, efficacy derived only from the words themselves; other times it also depended on the substances used for writing and on the material support of the text. It is possible that the practice of graphophagy reached medieval Europe from the ancient Mediterranean and the Middle East, a trajectory that highlights the continuity of such remedies well into Christian contexts.[49]

The analysis of ingested formulae across different regions and genres further demonstrates that what is often hastily classified as a "charm" (*carmen*) could be associated with a wide range of practitioners.[50] Graphophagic practices reveal substantial overlap between so-called "little" and "great" traditions, suggesting that such remedies were not confined to popular healers or marginal figures. As Robert Bjork has observed, the very fact that charms were written down implies that they were regarded as effective, not unlike prayers.[51] As Arnovick puts it, "what is sung or said or written in charms is as important a medicine as the botanical compounds made from charm recipes."[52]

Christianity played a crucial role in the transmission of charms from antiquity to the medieval world. Through Marcellus Empiricus and the manuscript

---

transkulturelle Perspektiven, ed. Carina Kühne-Wespi, Klaus Peter Oschema, and Joachim Friedrich Quack (de Gruyter, 2019), 359–72.

49 On this, with specific attention to textual amulets, see: Waldemar Deonna, "Abra, Abraca: La croix-talisman de Lausanne," *Genava* 22 (1944): 116–37; Jean Marquès-Rivière, *Amulettes, talismans et pentacles dans les traditions orientales et occidentales* (Payot, 1972); Marie-Thérèse d'Alverny, "Survivance de la magie antique," in *Antike und Orient im Mittelalter: Vorträge der Kölner Mediävistentagungen, 1956–1959*, ed. Paul Wilpert, Miscellanea Mediaevalia, Veröffentlichungen des Thomas-Instituts an der Universität Köln, vol. 1 (De Gruyter, 1962), 154–78; Alfons A. Barb, "The Survival of Magic Arts," in *The Conflict Between Paganism and Christianity in the Fourth Century*, ed. Arnaldo Momigliano (Clarendon Press, 1963), 100–25.

50 For an analysis of the notion of "charm," see Skemer, *Binding Words*, 9–14; Suzanne Sheldon Parnell and Lea T. Olsan, "The Index of Charms: Purpose, Design, and Implementation," *Literary and Linguistic Computing* 6, no. 1 (1991): 59–63, at 59. Within a medieval context, this term could refer to both oral and written words that were attributed specific powers.

51 Robert Bjork, ed. and trans., *Old English Shorter Poems. Vol. 2. Wisdom and Lyric* (University Press for Dumbarton Oaks Medieval Library, 2014), ix.

52 Arnovick, *Verbal Medicines*, 4. On the difference between written records and oral performances of charms, see: Lea T. Olsan, "Latin Charms of Medieval England: Verbal Healing in a Christian Oral Tradition," *Oral Tradition* 7, no. 1 (1992): 116–42; Lori Ann Garner, "Anglo-Saxon Charms in Performance," *Oral Tradition* 19, no. 1 (2004): 20–42; Stephen A. Mitchell, "Anaphrodisiac Charms in the Nordic Middle Ages: Impotence, Infertility, and Magic," *Norveg* 38 (1998): 19–42.

tradition of the *Physica Plinii*, charms were adapted to the cultural and religious framework of Christian Europe.[53] Along this same trajectory, however, charms intended for ingestion remained marginal – sometimes quite literally so, as they occasionally appear in the margins of manuscript folios. This book seeks to understand if such remedies were perceived as categorically different from more conventional charms, and whether their marginal status derived from the unusual and potentially transgressive nature of their mode of use.

Finally, this study brings into dialogue two fields that have rarely intersected: the history of food and the history of magic. Food historians have traditionally focused on conviviality, exchange, trade, taste, identity, and culinary practices, while historians of magic have concentrated on legislation, material culture, ritual performance, and cosmology.[54] Interactions between these two micro-fields of study have been sporadic and have yet to realise their full potential. For instance, Piero Camporesi explored food's magical and occult dimensions and its use as a medium of sympathetic magic in rural and early modern contexts.[55] Alban Gautier has analysed the medical and magical uses of food in Anglo-Saxon leechbooks, encouraging further research on food in such contexts.[56] The consumption of food and beverages believed to convey special virtues has been documented in countless sources from antiquity to modern times, although the topic has not been particularly fashionable in recent scholarship.[57]

---

53 Lea T. Olsan, "Charms in Late Antiquity and Early Medieval Medicine: Transmission and Transformation," in *Early Medieval Medicine in Context. Transmission, Translation and Transformation*, ed. Debby Banham, Claire Burridge, and Lea T. Olsan (Boydell&Brewer, 2025), 166–204, at 192ff.

54 A recent summary of the relevant bibliography is provided in Andrea Maraschi, "Anthropophagy and Graphophagy in Medieval Scandinavia. Magic, Boundaries, and New Methodological Approaches to Food History," in *Entangled Food Histories. Methods and Sources for Exploring Foodways across Millennia*, ed. Giacomo Casucci, Sofia Miola, Pietro Repishti and Sara Zanotta (Edizioni dell'Orso, 2025), 101–32, at 101–2.

55 Piero Camporesi, *Il pane selvaggio* (il Mulino, 1980); Id., *La carne impassibile* (il Saggiatore, 1983); Id., *Il sugo della vita: simbolismo e magia del sangue* (Mondadori, 1988); Id., *La terra e la luna: alimentazione, folclore, società* (il Saggiatore, 1989).

56 Alban Gautier, "Entre cuisine, médecine et magie : l'historien de l'alimentation face à quelques textes anglo-saxons," *Revue belge de Philologie et d'Histoire* 93, no. 2 (2015): 287–302.

57 E.g.: Frank M. Dugan, "Seldom Just Food: Garlic in Magic and Medicine in European and Mediterranean Traditions," *Digest: A Journal of Foodways and Culture* 5, no. 1 (2016): 1–60; Annie Thwaite, "What Is a 'Witch-Bottle'? Assembling the Textual Evidence from Early Modern England," *Magic, Ritual, and Witchcraft* 15, no. 2 (2020): 227–51; Andrea Maraschi, "Episodes of Cannibalism between Christians and Muslims from the Eleventh to the Thirteenth Centuries. Cases of Dehumanization and Hyper-Humanization," *Food, Culture*

There are many reasons why food-related topics should be relevant to historians of magic, and why investigations into techniques and ideas related to magic should interest food historians. One of the most important reasons concerns identity, as food shapes the eater's identity.[58] Similarly, practitioners of rituals addressed as *magic* also possessed distinct identities that varied over time and across regions, yet were grounded in a strong sense of rationality and experiential knowledge.[59]

•••

Taking these considerations into account, this monograph aims to study the use of written and, secondarily, spoken formulae in connection with acts of ingestion, analysing how words were thought to act upon reality and nature. The texts containing such formulae were not intended for reading in the modern sense, except in particular circumstances. Their circulation was often restricted to small and specific groups: practitioners, patients, clerics, or healers. In some cases, the formulae were copied without being fully understood, preserved because an authoritative tradition conferred value and efficacy upon them. In other cases, they were neither comprehended by those who uttered them nor by those who ingested them. However, their power was independent of this. Written in ancient and/or authoritative languages such as Hebrew, Greek, or Latin, as well as in vernacular languages, words and formulae represent central references throughout the Middle Ages in medical, ritual, and devotional practices.[60] It will become apparent that, in our sources, words are never utilised thoughtlessly. Even though they might have been more readily available than other medicinal ingredients, particular formulae were carefully

---

& Society (2024): https://doi.org/10.1080/15528014.2023.2300100; Karolina Tomczyszyn, "'Anoint Your Chest and Eat Some of the Wax-Salve:' The Non-Liturgical Use of Holy Oils in the Early Byzantine East," *Greek, Roman, and Byzantine Studies* 63 (2023): 325–49.

58 Peter Scholliers, "Meals, Food Narratives, and Sentiments of Belonging in Past and Present," in *Food, Drink and Identity. Cooking, Eating and Drinking in Europe Since the Middle Ages*, ed. Peter Scholliers (Berg, 2001), 3–22, at 3–4.

59 Harold Remus, "'Magic,' Method, Madness," *Method & Theory in the Study of Religion* 11, no. 3 (1999): 258–98; Bernd-Christian Otto, *Magie. Rezeptions- und diskursgeschichtliche Analysen von der Antike bis zur Neuzeit* (de Gruyter, 2011); Id., "Historicising 'Western Learned Magic:' Preliminary Remarks," *Aries* 16, no. 2 (2016): 161–240; Theodore S. de Bruyn, *Making Amulets Christian: Artefacts, Scribes, and Contexts* (Oxford University Press, 2017), 14–16.

60 On knowledge of Greek, see for example Joseph Rawson Lumby, *Greek Learning in the Western Church during the Seventh and Eighth Centuries, A.D.* (Cambridge, 1878).

selected and administered. Their repetition, material form, and – at times – their "dosage" were understood as essential to the activation of their power.

For medieval actors, the notion of "consuming" texts – whether through recitation or ingestion – was not inherently problematic, despite its strangeness from a modern perspective.[61] The Hippocratic-Galenic model of medicine offered a systematic framework for understanding the body's functions, mitigating some fears about health. However, its prescribed treatments were often both painful and ineffective. In contrast, talismans, ritual objects, and potions empowered by spoken or written incantations were generally harmless and, at the very least, consolatory. These remedies could operate as potent placebos, offering relief without the negative effects of more invasive interventions.[62] Psychological research suggests that humans have a natural tendency to attribute agency to unseen forces and to favour belief over evidence when confronting uncertainty,[63] a disposition that may offer evolutionary advantages in managing anxiety.[64] While such findings cannot be projected uncritically onto medieval contexts, they help to explain the appeal and persistence of ritualised practices such as graphophagy.

The analysis that follows is based on a substantial corpus of manuscripts and edited sources from western and northern Europe and is organised geographically, in order to reconstruct patterns of diffusion and circulation. The focus on the early and high medieval West reflects both the relative scarcity of sources and the limited attention this material has received from previous scholarship. The study does not extend beyond the twelfth century, except for brief comparative remarks, because the large-scale transmission of Arabic

61 I write "orally" since oral formulas were sometimes recited as a food or drink were being ingested.

62 Arthur K. Shapiro and Elaine Shapiro, *The Powerful Placebo. From Ancient Priest to Modern Physician* (The Johns Hopkins University Press, 1997), 53; Margaret Healy, "Wearing powerful words and objects: healing prosthetics," *Textual Practice* 30, no. 7 (2016): 1233–51; Dinesh Bhugra and Antonio Ventriglio, "Do Cultures Influence Placebo Response?," *Acta Psychiatrica Scandinavica* 132, no. 4 (2015): 227–30; Fabrizio Benedetti, Alessandro Piedimonte, and Elisa Frisaldi, "How Do Placebos Work?," *European Journal of Psychotraumatology* 9, sup3 (2018): https://doi.org/10.1080/2.

63 Christine Mohr, Lise Lesaffre, and Gustav Kuhn, "Magical Potential: Why Magic Performances Should be Used to Explore the Psychological Factors Contributing to Human Belief Formation," *Integrative Psychological and Behavioral Science* 53 (2019): 126–37; Paul Bloom, "Religion Is Natural," *Developmental Science* 10, 1 (2007): 147–51; Pascal Boyer, "Being Human. Religion: Bound to Believe?," *Nature* 455 (2008): 1038–39.

64 C. Harry Hui, Sing-Hang Cheung, Jasmine Lam, Esther Yuet Ying Lau, Livia Yuliawati, and Shu Fai Cheung, "In Search of the Psychological Antecedents and Consequences of Christian Conversion: A Three-Year Prospective Study," *Psychology of Religion and Spirituality* 9, no. 2 (2017): 220–30.

scientific and philosophical texts into Latin fundamentally reshaped learned conceptions of nature, causality, and magic. This process – often described as part of the "twelfth-century Renaissance" – introduced new theoretical frameworks, including the notion of natural magic as a legitimate field of inquiry, even as suspicions of demonic involvement persisted.

It is in this context that texts such as the *De radiis stellarum* (also known as the *Theorica artium magicarum*), long attributed to Abū Yūsuf Yaʿqūb al-Kindī (*c.*801–873),[65] circulated widely in Latin translation. The treatise articulated a theory of the natural efficacy of words and sounds, understood as endowed with power by the structure of the cosmos itself, regardless of semantic meaning. What mattered was correct utterance, solemnity, and intention – principles that resonate with earlier and less systematised assumptions about verbal efficacy found in graphophagic practices.[66]

Graphophagy offers a privileged vantage point from which to observe broader dynamics: the permeability of boundaries between medicine, devotion, and ritual; the authority attributed to written and spoken formulae; and the ways in which people acted upon uncertainty, illness, and desire. Why were certain texts eaten rather than read or spoken? How were words thought to operate once internalised? And what does the persistence of such practices reveal about medieval cultures of efficacy?

These are some of the questions at the heart of this book.

65 On this attribution, see Sylvain Matton, "An Irradiation of Latin Grammarians, or The *De radiis* Is Not by al-Kindī," *Magic, Ritual, and Witchcraft* 17, no. 3 (2022): 437–55.

66 Ya'Qub Ibn Ishaq al-Kindi, *De radiis. Teorica delle arti magiche. Un trattato medievale di magia naturale e astrologia fondamentale per l'Islam e l'Occidente*, ed. Ezio Abrile and Stefano Fumagalli, trans. Emanuela Turri (Mimesis, 2014 [1994]), 77.

CHAPTER 1

Words from Late Antiquity

An inquiry into the practice of ingesting written words and formulae must consider the extralinguistic power attributed to language.[1] This power manifests in rituals involving recitation of formulae, manipulation of objects, and use of specific substances or plants – practices regarded as efficacious even when they failed, since they addressed practical outcomes rather than abstract understanding.[2] Writing functioned as a practical technology within ritual contexts. Textual amulets, for instance, were widespread precisely because written texts were seen as durable embodiments of power.

Consequently, any attempt to account for the association between language and power must begin by addressing its underlying rationale. In many religious traditions, the act of creation itself is effected through a single word uttered by a deity. Ritual-linguistic operations can be categorised into three types: fiatic, Orphic, and talismanic. Fiatic operations refer the creation of the signified through the signifier, exemplifying the concept of bringing of the world into being through the λόγος. The Orphic category encompasses the capacity to influence an entity through vocal expression. Talismanic operations, by contrast, involve the ability to attract or channel power by means of language.[3] A fundamental assumption underlying such practices is that a word is equivalent to the thing it names, that the signifier coincides with its signified – although certain languages have traditionally been regarded as intrinsically more powerful than others, notably ancient or foreign tongues, and learned languages rather than the vernacular.[4] The signifiers employed in invocations, conjurations, consecrations, and similar acts are therefore seen as forms of performative language, a notion articulated by scholars such as Tambiah and Austin, who argue that utterances are intended to effect change in the world rather than merely convey information.[5] In other terms, to utter is to act.[6]

---

1 On the powers of spoken words, see for instance: Burnett, "The Theory and Practice of Powerful Words"; Delaurenti, *La Puissance des mots.*

2 William Sax, Johannes Quack, and Jan Weinhold, ed., *The Problem of Ritual Efficacy* (Oxford University Press, 2010).

3 Moshe Idel, "On Talismanic Language in Jewish Mysticism," *Diogenes* 43, no. 2 (1995): 23–41.

4 Malinowski, *Coral Gardens*, II, 213–22.

5 Stanley J. Tambiah, *Culture, Thought and Social Action* (Harvard University Press, 1985).

6 Austin, *How to Do Things With Words*, 6–7.

 | HTTPS://DOI.ORG/10.1163/9789004765528-003

This principle was often employed in magic books and texts circulating widely throughout the eastern Mediterranean.[7] Coptic and Graeco-Egyptian papyri constitute some of the most significant surviving evidence of this tradition, while the early Christian Church devoted considerable effort to identifying and prohibiting comparable works, which it associated with paganism and idolatry.[8] The same attitude had already been set in the Torah, where the practices of *malefici*, *incantatores*, *pythones* and *divini* are considered abominations (Deut 18:9–12).[9]

Graphophagy, in particular, has a long and documented history in the Mediterranean world, which predates Christianity and provides an essential backdrop for its medieval manifestations. In ancient Egypt, inscribed stelae featuring hieroglyphs and images were believed to possess specific powers: water poured over them was often consumed for protective purposes, illustrating the integration of written language with ritual efficacy.[10] The ingestion of written text also appears in the first tale of Setne Khamwas (Cairo CG 30646, *c.* third century BCE), where knowledge contained in the god Thoth's book is acquired by copying it onto papyrus, dissolving the sheets in beer and water, and drinking the mixture.[11] Related assumptions underlie the "Cannibal Hymn" of the Pyramid Texts, which implies that the divine force may be literally absorbed

7 Owen Davies, *Grimoires: A History of Magic Books* (Oxford University Press, 2009), 18.

8 Jacco Dieleman, "The Greco-Egyptian Magical Papyri," in *Guide to the Study of Ancient Magic*, ed. David Frankfurter (Brill, 2019), 283–321, esp. 283–4; Valerie I.J. Flint, "The Demonisation of Magic and Sorcery in Late Antiquity: Christian Redefinitions of Pagan Religions," in *Magic and Witchcraft in Ancient Europe*, vol. II: *Ancient Greece and Rome*, ed. Bengt Ankarloo and Stuart Clark (University of Pennsylvania Press, 1999), 279–348. See for instance Clayton N. Jefford, *Didache. The Teaching of the Twelve Apostles* (Polebridge Press, 2013), iii.4, 25, and v.1, 31.

9 Brian B. Schmidt, "Canaanite Magic vs. Israelite Religion: Deuteronomy 18 and the Taxonomy of Taboo," in *Magic and Ritual in the Ancient World*, ed. Paul Mirecki and Marvin Meyer (Brill, 2002), 242–59; Stephen D. Ricks, "The Magician as Outsider in the Hebrew Bible and the New Testament," in *Ancient Magic and Ritual Power*, 131–43, at 137–8. The New Testament endorsed such position, as in Gal 5:21 and Rev 21:8.

10 Pierre Lacau, "Les statues 'guérisseuses' dans l'ancienne Egypte," *Académie des inscriptions et belles-lettres. Commission de la fondation Poit, Monuments et Mémoires* 25 (1921–22): 189–209; Francisco Marco Simón, "Materiality, Oral Incantations and Supernatural Agency in Ancient Healing Magic," *Acta Classica Universitatis Scientiarum Debreceniensis* 57 (2021): 15–42, at 19.

11 Koering, *Iconophages*, 160–2; Frankfurter, "The Magic of Writing," 634–5. See also *Héros, magiciens et sages oubliés de l'Égypte ancienne: Une anthologie de la littérature en égyptien démotique*, ed. Damien Agut-Mabordère and Michel Chauveau (Les Belles Lettres, 2011), 24–7.

through ingestion,[12] as well as Ptolemaic narratives in which scribes drink liquified books in order to internalise their power.[13] These examples reflect a widely shared belief system rather than isolated practices, transcending literacy levels and indicating a rich tradition where writing was understood as materially efficacious across various cultures such as Christianity, Islam, and Buddhism, all of which developed sophisticated ideologies attributing power to texts, books, and writing surfaces.[14] Thus, medieval graphophagy should not be viewed as an anomaly but rather as a continuation of a much older and pervasive tendency to anchor supernatural efficacy in material practices.

Aristotle maintained that "spoken words are the symbols of mental experience and written words are the symbols of spoken words."[15] This implies that, in his view, *phōnē* (φωνή), that is spoken language, is not arbitrary but gives expression to internal thoughts and mental states, since language is rooted in the *psychē* (ψυχή), the soul. Speech is therefore the means by which human beings symbolise and communicate the contents of their thoughts and experiences. Writing (*grammata*, γράμματα), in turn, constitutes a visual representation of spoken words. It stands at one further remove from thought, yet it captures and fixes it in visible form. This conceptual framework helps to explain why words, phrases, and formulae were regarded as fully capable of transmitting powers or triggering effects when ink and writing surfaces were ingested. Yet, in ritual practices writing could become detached from actual thoughts, or at least the connection between thought and visual sign could become obscure.[16] Medieval philosophers such as Augustine, Boethius, and Anselm of Canterbury engaged the question of whether both written and spoken words derived from mental concepts that were naturally similar across all humans. Such ideas allowed writing to participate, however indirectly, in universal rational structure and created conceptual space for graphophagic efficacy, at least in theory.[17]

---

12 *The Cannibal Hymn*, in *Writings from Ancient Egypt*, trans. Toby Wilkinson (Penguin, 2016), 89–92.

13 Simón, "Materiality, Oral Incantations and Supernatural Agency," 20.

14 Frankfurter, "The Magic of Writing in Mediterranean Antiquity."

15 Arist., *Int.*, 1.16a3–4.

16 Linda E. Voigts, "The Character of the Carecter: Ambiguous Sigils in Scientific and Medical Texts," in *Latin and Vernacular: Studies in Late-Medieval Texts and Manuscripts*, ed. Alastair J. Minnis (D.S. Brewer, 1989), 91–109; Benoît Grévin and Julien Véronèse, "Les 'caractères' magiques au Moyen Age (XIIe–XIVe siècle)," *Bibliothèque de l'École des Chartres* 162 (2004): 305–79.

17 David K. Coley, *The Wheel of Language. Representing Speech in Middle English Poetry, 1377–1422* (Syracuse University Press, 2012), 35–6; Luisa Valente, "*Verbum mentis – Vox clamantis*: The Notion of the Mental Word in Twelfth-Century Theology," in *The Word in Medieval*

Numerous instances of so-called "magical gibberish" – unconventional script patterns and inventive graphic solutions – highlight the diverse ways in which writing was utilised within ritual contexts, emphasising its symbolic and performative dimensions. Pliny the Elder's ambivalence towards what he termed *magicae vanitates* highlights a critical tension in the perception of written language within Roman society. While he questioned the intrinsic power of words, his accounts reflect a broader cultural scepticism about the efficacy of magical texts: "The greatest and ever uncertain question concerning remedies derived from humans is whether words and incantations of charms have any power," Pliny writes.[18] If words did possess such power, all mankind would indeed have reason to be grateful. Yet, Pliny adds, the wisest men rejected this belief, in contrast to the illiterate.

The use of writing in ritual contexts catalysed the reinvention of the purpose and value of this technology, from special script patterns to the implementation of *voces magicae* – incomprehensible or non-natural sequences of letters or obscure words – and coded *charaktêres*.[19] As observed by David Frankfurter, within such contexts the written word is characterised by an ambiguity "between image and semantic sign," and the writing surface by an ambiguity "between vehicle of communication and vehicle impregnated with the power of the written (or spoken) word."[20] By and large, scholarship has been able to cast light on a broad Mediterranean culture of ritual writing attested from the Hellenistic period through Late Antiquity, and deeply rooted in Egyptian and Jewish cultures, among others.

Logic, Theology and Psychology. Acts of the XIII International Colloquium of the Société Internationale pour l'étude de la Philosophie Médiévale, Kyoto, 27 September–1 October 2005 (Brepols, 2009), 365–402.

18 Pliny the Elder, *Naturalis Historia libri XXXVII*, ed. Karl F.T. Mayhoff (Teubner, 1906), xxviii, 10: "Ex homine remediorum primum maximae quaestionis et semper incertae est, polleantne aliquid verba et incantamenta carminum. Quod si verum est, homini acceptum fieri oportere conveniat; sed viritim sapientissimi cuiusque respuit fides, in universum vero omnibus horis credit vita nec sentit." On this, see Maraschi, Similia similibus curantur, 37–42.

19 Henk Versnel, "The Poetics of the Magical Charm: An Essay in the Power of Words," in *Magic and Ritual in the Ancient World*, 105–56; Magali de Haro Sanchez, ed., *Écrire la magie dans l'antiquité : Actes du colloque international (Liège, 13–15 octobre 2011)* (Presses Universitaires de Liège, 2015); Richard Gordon, "*Charaktēres* between Antiquity and Renaissance: Transmission and Re-Invention," in *Les savoirs magiques et leur transmission de l'antiquité à la Renaissance*, ed. Véronique Dasen and Jean-Michel Spieser (SISMEL – Edizioni del Galluzzo, 2014), 253–300; Richard Gordon, "From Substance to Text: Three Materialities of 'Magic' in the Roman Imperial Period," in *The Materiality of Magic*, ed. Dietrich Boschung and Jan N. Bremmer (Wilhlem Fink, 2015), 133–76.

20 Frankfurter, "The Magic of Writing in Mediterranean Antiquity," 627.

For what concerns the Bible and Jewish tradition, evidence of the powers attributed to words and to practices of graphophagy may not be abundant, but requires careful attention because it reveals how textual consumption could be rendered theologically legitimate through scriptural precedent.[21] The idea that knowledge could be ingested, as for the apple in Gn 3:5–7, was deeply rooted in this tradition.[22] Perhaps the two best known biblical references to graphophagy are in the Book of Ezekiel and in the Book of Revelation.[23] In Ezekiel 2:8–3:3, Yahweh commands the Israelite priest to consume – literally, to devour[24] – a scroll, showing the profound connection between the act of ingestion and the internalisation of divine authority. It is a call from God to be a prophet to Israel during the critical time of the Babylonian exile.[25] To speak to the rebellious nation of Israel, God gives Ezekiel a scroll to eat ("aperi os tuum et comede quaecumque ego do tibi," "open your mouth and eat what I give you"),[26] which allows him to internalise Yahweh's words. The scroll "erat scriptus intus et foris et scriptae erant in eo lamentationes et carmen et vae" ("on both sides of it were written words of lament and mourning and woe"), indicating the harsh nature of the message Ezekiel was to deliver.[27] Despite its bitter contents, however, the scroll tastes "sicut mel dulce" ("as sweet as honey"),[28] the typical flavour of God in Jewish-Christian tradition.[29] A strong case could be made that these verses were just a metaphor for the mental and spiritual absorption of God's Word by Ezekiel.[30]

The passage can be understood along the lines of a similar – earlier – call to prophecy to Jeremiah, during the early stages of the Babylonian exile.

---

21 Joshua Trachtenberg, *Jewish Magic and Superstition: A Study in Folk Religion* (The University of Pennsylvania Press, 1939), 122–24.

22 Mark S. Smith, "Evil in Genesis and Other Ancient Near Eastern Creation Stories," in *Narrating the Beginnings*, ed. Alberto Bernabé Pajares and Raquel Martín Hernández (Springer, 2021), 95–116, at 104.

23 Biblical quotations are from *Biblia Sacra Vulgata*, ed. Robert Weber and Roger Gryson, 5th ed. (Deutsche Biblegesellschaft, 2007). Translation into English are from the New International Version (NIV).

24 Massimo Leone, "Le Dieu mâché. Idéologies du sens religieux et mastication." *Lexia. Rivista di semiotica* 19–20 (2015): 247–64, at 251–2.

25 Margaret S. Odell, "You Are What You Eat: Ezekiel and the Scroll," *Journal of Biblical Literature* 117, no. 2 (1998): 229–48, at 241–45.

26 Ez 2:8.

27 Ez 2:10.

28 Ez 3:3.

29 Rachel F. Brown, "'Taste and See That the Lord is Sweet' (Ps. 33:9): The Flavor of God in the Monastic West," *The Journal of Religion* 86, no. 2 (2006): 169–204.

30 Caroline Walker Bynum, *Holy Feast and Holy Fast: The Religious Significance of Food to Medieval Women* (University of California Press, 1990), 150.

Here, God symbolically touches Jeremiah's mouth, empowering him to speak on God's behalf.[31] What is more, Ezekiel's act of graphophagy (which is also hierophagy)[32] inspired a scene in the Book of Revelation where John of Patmos is instructed by a voice from heaven to take a small scroll from the hand of an angel. He is told to eat the scroll, which tastes sweet in his mouth but turns bitter in his stomach – symbolising the sweetness of divine revelation and the bitterness of God's judgments. After consuming it, John is told that he must prophesy again about peoples, nations, languages, and kings.[33] This passage can be similarly interpreted metaphorically as a way to describe how humans could access the divine realm by consuming otherwordly items.[34] This approach is further encouraged by verses such as Ps 118:103, where the psalmist celebrates the beauty, power, and sweetness of God's commandments and teachings and expresses a deep personal affection for God's word.

When Jerome comments on Ezekiel's scroll consumption, he emphasises that "when, through assiduous meditation, we have stored the book of the Lord in the treasury of memory, our belly is spiritually filled and our inner parts are satisfied."[35] Similarly, Augustine holds that consuming scripture means internalising its teaching through meditative rumination.[36]

However, a purely metaphorical interpretation may not suffice to account fully for Ezekiel's and John's ingestion of the scroll. It has been suggested that the eating act may be connected with the ordeal described in Num 5, yet this line of interpretation has largely foregrounded symbolic resonances rather than its practical dimensions.[37] Nevertheless, the cultural power attributed to written letters should not be underestimated.[38] In the Book of Numbers one

---

31 Jer 1:9.

32 From hieros, ἱερός, "sacred," "holy," the act of consuming some otherwordly item. There are several examples of the consumption of otherwordly foods and items in classical literature. In some cases, the act of consumption results in the acquisition of divine knowledge.

33 Rev 10:10. See Craig R. Koester, *Revelation: A New Translation with Introduction and Commentary* (Yale University Press, 2014), 482.

34 For instance, see Meredith J.C. Warren, "Tasting the Little Scroll: A Sensory Analysis of Divine Interaction in Revelation 10.8–10," *Journal for the Study of the New Testament* 40, no. 1 (2017): 101–19.

35 Jerome, *Commentariorum in Hiezechielem libri XIV*, ed. Francisco Glorie, CCSL 75 (Brepols, 1964), 3–743, 1.3.

36 Namely in his *Contra Faustum* about Manicheans: Andrea Piras, *Verba lucis. Scrittura, immagine e libro nel manicheismo* (Mimesis, 2012), 79–80 and n. 101.

37 Moshe Greenberg, *Ezekiel 1–20: A New Translation with Introduction and Commentari* (Doubleday, 1983), 78.

38 Nili Shupak, "'Eat This Scroll' (Ezekiel 3:1): Writing as Symbol and Metaphor in the Hebrew Bible in the Light of Ancient Near Eastern Sources," *Bibliotheca Orientalis* 70,

encounters the description of the *sotah* ritual – the ordeal of the bitter water – which provides differently configured but equally important precedent.[39] In this context, the ingestion of words is not metaphorical at all, but constitutes a concrete ritual act. This practice would later provide Christians with a legal and conceptual precedent for the ritual use of liquids believed to possess supernatural efficacy.[40] This ritual thus exemplifies the ways in which words were employed to produce effects that were materially tangible and publicly observable.[41]

The ordeal of the bitter water was intended to determine, through divine invocation, whether a wife had been unfaithful to her husband. The underlying principle of ordeals was that of a "trial" in which the divine judgement – God alone being capable of knowing the truth of an individual's guilt or innocence – would be made manifest.[42] This passage belongs to a section of the Book of Numbers that repeatedly addresses the purification of the Israelites and their camp, in accordance with the commands given by God to Moses.[43] This ordeal was designed to test a woman's fidelity when her husband suspected adultery but lacked evidence, a situation that undermined the stability of the household and, by extension, of the wider community.[44] Most strikingly, the procedure involved an act of graphophagy. The woman was brought before a priest, who mixed holy water with dust taken from the floor of the tabernacle and wrote a curse on parchment, which was then dissolved in the water. The woman was required to drink this mixture and, if she were guilty, the curse was believed to produce physical afflictions: her abdomen would swell and her thighs would waste away – a phrase alternatively translated as referring to the collapse or

no. 1–2 (2013): 25–41, at 33–37; Gerald A. Klingbeil, "'Eating' and 'Drinking' in the Book of Revelation: A Study of New Testament Thought and Theology," *Journal of the Adventist Theological Society* 16, no. 1–2 (2005): 75–92.

39 Num 5:11–31. The description also appears in Prot. Jas. 16:2 (II century).

40 On this, see Tikva Frymer-Kensky, "The Strange Case of the Suspected Sotah (Numbers v 11–31)," *Vetus Testamentum* no. 34 (1984): 11–26.

41 Naomi Janowitz, "Water, Word and Name: The Shifting Pragmatics of the Sotah/Suspected Adulteress Ritual," in *Literature or Liturgy ? Early Christian Hymns and Prayers in their Literary and Liturgical Context in Antiquity*, ed. Clemens Leonhard and Hermut Löhr (Mohr Siebeck, 2014), 15–31.

42 Daniel Friedmann, *Diritto e morale nelle storie bibliche*, trans. Diana Zerilli (Giuffrè Editore, 2008), 37ff.

43 Marina Lalatta Costerbosa, "Per una storia critica della tortura," *Materiali per una storia della cultura giuridica* 1 (2011): 3–34; Eve L. Feinstein, "The 'Bitter Waters' of Numbers 5:11–31," *Vetus Testamentum* 62 (2012): 300–306.

44 Walter C. Kaiser, *Toward Old Testament Ethics* (Zondervan, 1983), 223–30.

discharge of the genital tract[45] – thus revealing her unfaithfulness.[46] If the woman were pregnant, the "bitter water" would induce miscarriage and cause further complications, such as abdominal swelling and sterility. An innocent woman, by contrast, would remain unaffected.

Might the effects have been linked to the way the ink was produced? Ink was commonly made from organic substances such as soot or carbon black mixed with water and gum Arabic.[47] In later periods, however, inks were increasingly produced from gall nuts (rich in tannins) combined with vitriol, which may account for the reference to bitterness.[48] Although such compounds could plausibly have produced physiological effects, it has been argued that the ordeal should not be explained primarily in pharmacological terms, but rather through psychological mechanisms. From this perspective, this ritual illustrates how the powers attributed to language contributed to the social construction of reality.[49] That said, some scholars have suggested that the "bitter water" may in fact have functioned as a potent abortifacient, possibly made from plants such as *Artemisia* and willow bark.[50]

Do the biblical narratives mentioned above and this Jewish ordeal offer any indication as to the practice of ingesting text? Medieval exegetes drew a clear

45 Charles J. Brim, *Medicine in the Bible* (Froben Press, 1936), 374.

46 On medieval interpretations of this text, see: Finbarr McAuley, "Canon Law and the End of the Ordeal," *Oxford Journal of Legal Studies* 26, 3 (2006): 473–513. On ordeals in Jewish tradition, see Shlomo Eidelberg, "Trial by Ordeal in Medieval Jewish History: Laws, Customs and Attitudes," in *Proceedings of the American Academy for Jewish Research*, vols. 46/47, Jubilee Volume (1928–29/1978–79), Part 1 (1979–1980), 105–20; Ronald B. Allen, "Numbers," in *The Expositor's Bible Commentary: Genesis, Exodus, Leviticus, Numbers*, vol. 2, ed. Frank E. Gaebelein (Zondervan, 1990), 655–1008, at 743.

47 Robert Sobott, Nadine Quenouille, Reinhold Scholl, Klaus Bente, and Christoph Berthold, "Non-Destructive Studies on Ostraca Texts, Inks and Their Ceramic Substrates," in *Archäometrie und Denkmalpflege 2015: Jahrestagung an der Johannes Gutenberg-Universität Mainz, Metalla Sonderheft 7*, ed. T. Gluhak, S. Greiff, K. Kraus and M. Prange (Deutsches Bergbau-Museum, 2015), 248–50.

48 Christian Frevel, "On Instant Scripture and Proximal Texts: Some Insights into the Sensual Materiality of Texts and their Ritual Roles in the Hebrew Bible and Beyond," *Postscripts: The Journal of Sacred Texts, Cultural Histories, and Contemporary Contexts* 8, no. 1–2 (2017): 57–79.

49 Richard Bauman and Charles L. Briggs, "Poetics and Performance as Critical Perspectives on Language and Social Life," *Annual Review of Anthropology* 19 (1990): 59–89, at 60.

50 John M. Riddle, "Women's Medicines in Ancient Jewish Sources: Fertility Enhancers and Inhibiters," in *Disease in Babylonia*, ed. Irving L. Finkel and Markham J. Geller (Brill, 2007), 200–214; Fred Rosner, *Medicine in the Bible and the Talmud* (Yeshiva University Press, 1995), 239–47; Julius Preuss, *Biblical and Talmudic Medicine*, trans. Fred Rosner (Jason Aronson, 1993); Wilhelm Epstein, *Die Medizin im Alten Testament* (Ferdinand Enke, 1901), 136–7.

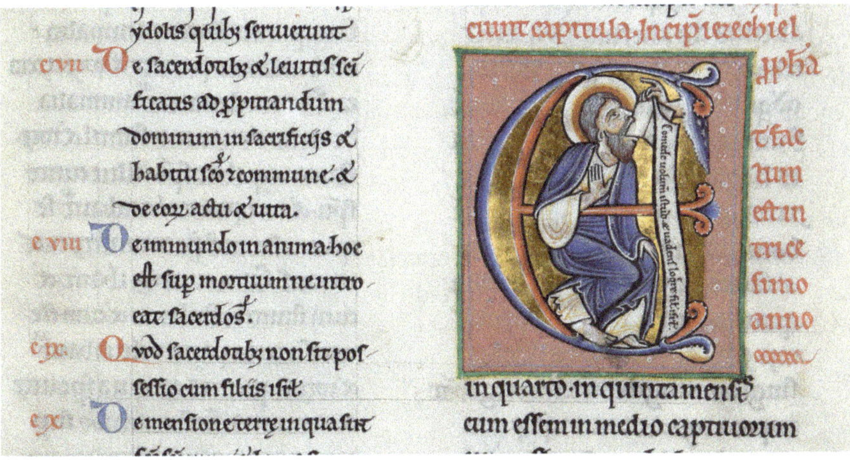

FIGURE 1 Ezekiel eats the bittersweet scroll containing a prophecy for the Israelites (illuminated initial E). Paris, BNF, MS Latin 16744, fol. 81r (Source: gallica.bnf.fr – Bibliothèque nationale de France)

distinction between the literal and the spiritual senses of Scripture, the latter comprising two or three subsidiary levels (tropological, allegorical and/or anagogical).[51] From this perspective, the act of chewing and digesting text symbolised the nourishment of the mind.[52] Yet medieval iconography persistently depicts the scenes of scroll consumption in the Book of Ezekiel and in the Revelation of John literally rather than metaphorically. In a Latin Bible dating from the second half of the twelfth century, an illuminated initial E shows Ezekiel in the act of eating the scroll (fig. 1).

The scroll clearly bears the inscription *comede volumen istud et vadens loquere ad filios Israel*: "eat this scroll; then go and speak to the people of Israel" (from Ez 3:1). This illuminated initial sits at the beginning of the Book of Ezekiel: *Et factum est in tricesimo anno* ("and it came to pass in the thirtieth year …"), the opening verse that establishes the setting for Ezekiel's prophetic ministry. The act of text consumption is thus the first image the reader engages with.

---

51 Robert E. McNally, "Medieval Exegesis," *Theological Studies* 22 (1961): 445–54; Frans van Liere, "Biblical Exegesis," in *Handbook of Medieval Studies. Terms – Methods – Trends*, ed. Albert Classen, 5 vols. (de Gruyter, 2010), vol. 1, 137–45, at 139.

52 Danielle Callegari, *Dante's Gluttons. Food and Society from the Convivio to the Comedy* (Amsterdam University Press, 2022), 53–4. See, for example, Gregory the Great's exegesis of Ezekiel's passage: Gregory the Great, *Homiliae in Hiezechihelem prophetam*, ed. Marcus Adriaen, CCSL 142 (Brepols, 1971), i.10. On the passage in Revelation, see Autpert Ambrose, *Expositio in Apocalypsin*, ed. Robert Weber, CCCM 27; 27A (Brepols, 1975), I, v.10.

Another striking example of an illuminated E at the onset of the Book of Ezekiel appears in the Lambeth Bible, dating from the mid-twelfth century. Here, the Israelite prophet is depicted twice: above, eating the scroll given to him by the hand of God, and below, holding a pot ink and a reed pen (fig. 2). Jérémie Koering suggests that the ink pot might have been wittingly placed at the level of Ezekiel's stomach, possibly alluding to the prophet's ingestion and incorporation of divine word.[53]

A comparable scene appears in an Apocalypse manuscript produced around 1255–1260, in which St. John is depicted chewing the book handed to him by an angel (fig. 3).

These visual representations may suggest that references to the ingestion of texts were, at least in some contexts, understood in a literal sense.[54] The images do not contradict allegorical readings but complement them: spiritual assimilation of God's word is real precisely because it can be materially enacted through consumption. This idea should not appear surprising, Massimo Leone observes, as Christianity had replaced the word of the Torah with the body of Christ, and placed the consumption of this body at the core of its ritual.[55] The metaphorical parallel between word and food was openly expressed in an influential commentary on the Gospel of Matthew dating from the fifth century, wrongly attributed to John Chrysostom. A passage about the opening section of Mt 22, which features the Parable of the Wedding Banquet, begins as follows: "Multas enim proprietates habet sermo ad escam" ("For speech has many properties similar to food").[56] Drawing on the analogy between spiritual and physical consumption, the exegete argues that the word of God requires a process of digestion: it must be examined (chewed), memorised (swallowed), and continuously recalled and meditated upon (ruminated). This digestive metaphor, which even invokes Mosaic dietary laws regarding clean animals that chew the cud, places memory and meditation as essential to spiritual nourishment and salvation.

53 Koering, *Iconophages*, 162.

54 Tsakos, "Materiality and Physicality of Medieval Manuscripts," 980. A further example is Jer 15:16. Here, the prophet laments the fate of Judah, who is facing increasing pressure from the Babylonian Empire, and struggles with his prophetic calling. God's judgment is imminent, having the people persistently sinned and rejected their covenant with him. Jeremiah has become a social outcast, and pleads with God for justice. By referring to an act of graphophagy, Jeremiah describes his deep internalisation of God's message, much like Ezekiel and John.

55 Leone, "Le Dieu mâché," 252–3.

56 *Eruditi commentarii in Evangelium Matthaei, incerto auctore*, in *Patrologiae cursus completus, series Graeca*, ed. Jacques-Paul Migne, 56 (Migne, 1862), 611–946, at 860. Cited in Leone, "Le Dieu mâché," 252–3.

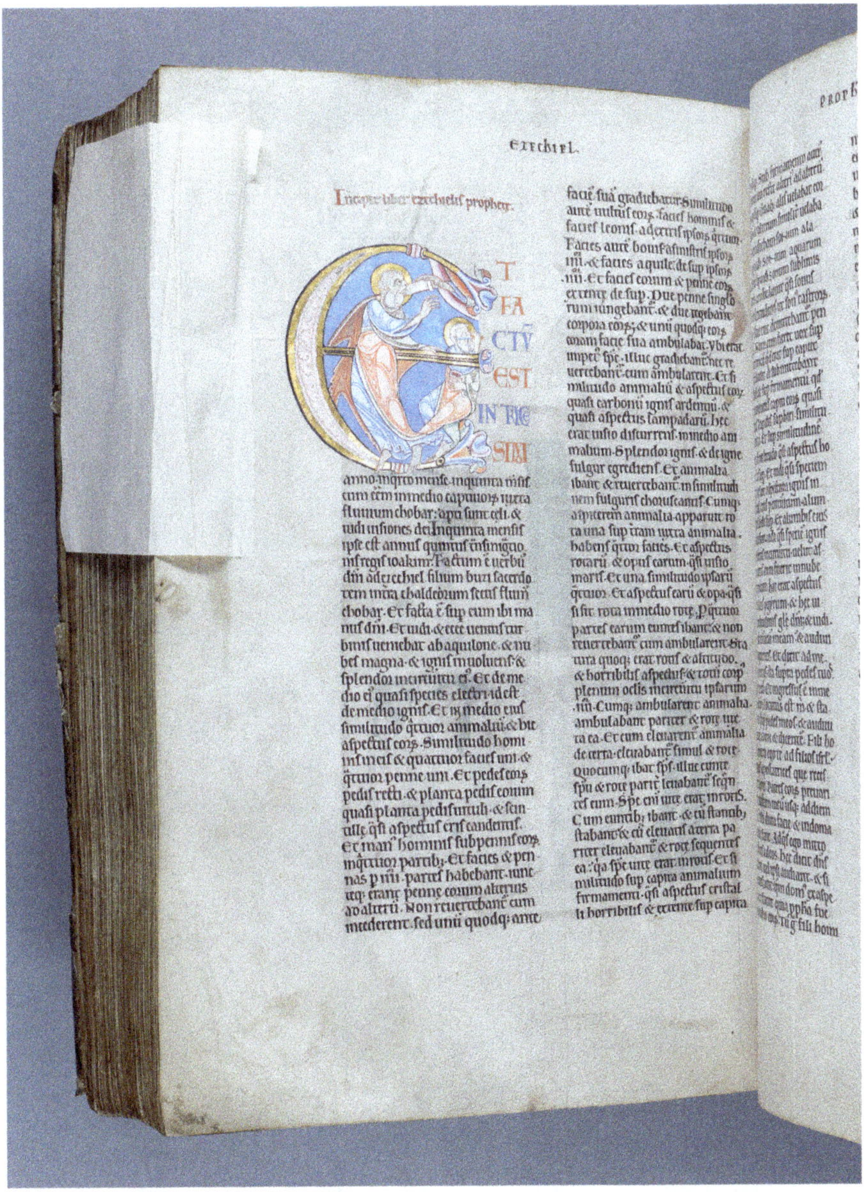

FIGURE 2 This illuminated initial E contains a double representation of Ezekiel: above, receiving and eating the scroll from the divine hand, and below, equipped with a pot of ink and a reed pen (*c.*1146). London, Lambeth Palace Library, MS 3, fol. 258v. Reproduced with permission of Lambeth Palace Library

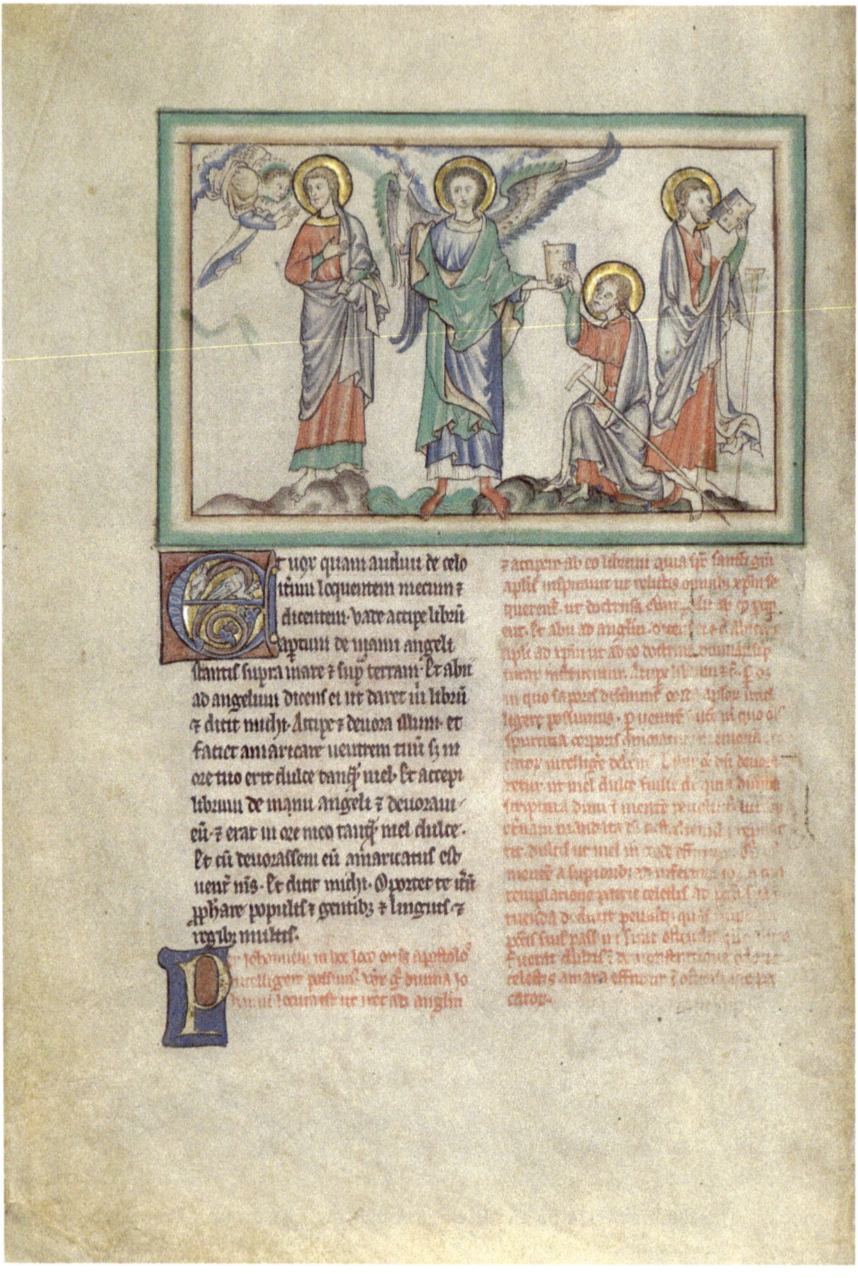

FIGURE 3 St. John eats the book received from the angel, about 1255–1260. Los Angeles, Getty Museum, Ludwig III 1 (83.MC.72), fol. 15v (Courtesy of Getty's Open Content Program)

This dual register – metaphorical meaning and literal enactment – appears characteristic of medieval textual culture more broadly. Monastic *ruminatio*[57] metaphorically compared reading to digestion while literally involving repetitive vocalisation that physically engaged the mouth and throat. Eucharistic theology insisted Christ's body was spiritually received yet materially consumed. Relic veneration maintained that saints' physical remains conveyed their sanctity while acknowledging that holiness transcended materiality. In each case, metaphorical interpretation coexisted with material practice rather than replacing it.

Evidence from both Western and Eastern cultures, well before the Middle Ages, suggests that the ingestion of letters and texts was believed to result in the assimilation of actual knowledge or information, or in the activation of powerful effects, such as the enhancement of memory.[58] Texts from the Cairo Genizah – that is, the vast collection of hundreds of thousands of manuscripts from the sixth century onwards preserved in the genizah of the Ben Ezra Synagogue – attest to rituals centred on the drinking of words, prayers, and other formulae, as well as on the washing of letters and divine names and the subsequent use of that water to knead cakes. Similarly, names or other formulae could be written on edible media, whether liquid (wine) or solid (figs, leaves, eggs). Similar practices are attested in rituals intended to "open one's heart" found in the Hekhalot literature, a corpus of Jewish esoteric texts dating from late antiquity and the Early Middle Ages. These prescriptions recommend writing names on a bowl, washing them off with water, and then drinking the liquid. Alternatively, the same water could be mixed with barley flour and used to prepare cakes, which were then consumed.[59]

At the same time, comparable practices also circulated within medical contexts. Around the early fifth century, a series of graphophagic remedies were recorded by Pseudo-Theodorus Priscianus. The treatise in which they appear was composed in the style of the near-contemporary medical writer Theodorus Priscianus, a pupil of Helvius Vindicianus, a fourth-century physician active

57 This idea stemmed from Lev 11:3: "omne quod habet divisam ungulam et ruminat in pecoribus comedetis." Shannon Gayk, "'Ete This Book:' Literary Consumption and Poetic Invention in Capgrave's Life of St. Katherine," in *Form and Reform. Reading across the Fifteenth Century*, ed. Shannon Gayk and Kathleen Tonry (Ohio State University Press, 2011), 88–109, esp. 95–99.

58 Michael D. Swartz, "Magical Piety in Ancient and Medieval Judaism," 178–9. See also Peter Schäfer, "Jewish Magic Literature in Late Antiquity and the Early Middle Ages," *Journal of Jewish Studies* 41 (1990): 75–91.

59 Schäfer, "Jewish Magic Literature," 90.

in northern Africa.[60] Although Theodorus' medical system was grounded in Hippocratic doctrine, Pseudo-Theodorus appears to have shown an interest in alternative therapeutic practices as well.[61] For the treatment of epistaxis, for instance, the following words were to be written on laurel leaves using the patient's blood: "Tantale pie, pie Tantale, Tantale pie," an invocation of the mythological figure Tantalus, condemned to eternal thirst in Tartarus.[62] The blood was then to be washed off with the juice of a young leek, and the resulting mixture given to the patient to drink. This example clearly suggests that analogical thinking and performative language constituted fundamental mechanisms underlying graphophagic remedies. The "thing" that was named coincided with the outcome to be achieved, even when the reference was metaphorical: internal thoughts took physical form and were believed to bring about physiological effects.

As we shall see, laurel leaves were often used as comfortable writing surfaces. Their strong aroma was associated with potent properties, widely employed in the eastern Mediterranean in divinatory practices, as natural protective amulets, to attract guardian spirits such as Christian angels or the pre-Islamic djinns, and to provoke sexual desire.[63] Indeed, botanical fragrances often reveal the presence of compounds with pharmacological effects, and for

---

60 Sadi Maréchal, *Public Baths and Bathing Habits in Late Antiquity. A Study of the Evidence from Italy, North Africa and Palestine A.D. 287–700* (Brill,2020), 40–1.

61 Alf Önnerfors, "Magische Formel nim Dienste römischer Medizin," in *Aufstieg und niedergang der römischen Welt*, ed. Wolfgang Haase and Hildegard Temporini, II, 37.1 (de Gruyter, 1993), 157–224.

62 Pseudo-Theodorus Priscianus, *Additamenta Pseudo-Theodori ad Theodorum Priscianum*, ed. Valentino Rose (Teubner, 1894), 276: "In tria folia lauri scribis de sanguine ipsius [qui patitur] 'Tantale pie, pie Tantale, Tantale pie,' et de suco porri virginis lavas folia ipsa, et da ei bibere." On the word "tantale," traditionally used to treat haemorrhages, see Alphonse A. Barb, "Bois du sang, Tantale," *Syria* 29, no. 3/4 (1952): 271–84; Christopher A. Faraone, "Does Tantalus Drink the Blood, or Not? An Enigmatic Series of Inscribed Hematite Gemstones," in *Antike Mythen Medien, Transformationen und Konstruktionen*, ed. Ueli Dill and Christine Walde (de Gruyter, 2009), 203–28.

63 Pliny the Elder, *Naturalis Historia*, xv.39–40.127–38; Isidoro di Siviglia, *Etimologie o origini*, ed. Angelo Valastro Canale, 2 vols. (UTET, 2013), II, 17.7.2. See, in the Greek Magical Papyri: PGM I.262–347; PGM II.1–64 e II.64–183; PGM III.282–409; PGM V.172–212; PGM VI.1–47; PGM VII.795–845 e 1009–16; PGM XIII.734–1077. The rituals to attract djinns and to arouse sexual appetite are in *Picatrix, Ghayat al-Hakim, The Goal of the Wise*, trans. From the Arabic by Hashem Atallah, 2 vols. (Ouroboros Press, 2002), II, 4–5, 238 and 242. In a ninth-century manuscript from northern Italy, an angel can be summoned through laurel leaves to treat headache: Uppsala, Universitetsbiblioteket C. 664, p. 176, viii. Martin of Braga mentions other pagan uses of laurel leaves: *De correctione rusticorum*, in *Martini Episcopi Bracarensis opera omnia*, ed. Claude W. Barlow (Yale University Press, 1950), 16, 198.

a long time humans relied on scent and taste to assess the safety, toxicity, and (un)desirable effects of natural ingredients.[64]

Another remedy suggested by Pseudo-Theodorus to induce sleep required now-incomprehensible words to be inscribed on the inside of a cup; the same words were also spoken into the vessel before the drink was administered to the insomniac patient.[65] For the same purpose, alternative prescriptions instructed that other words be incised on a ball – or possibly a short column – of wax and then heated or burned, the smoke being inhaled through the nose.[66]

This attitude is consistent with the rituals discussed above, which were practiced in Jewish milieux. The *Euporiston* of Theodorus Priscianus has survived in a Latin version, possibly produced by the author himself and abridged from a now-lost Greek original. Practical in character, the work circulated within the bilingual milieu of late antique North Africa and was conceived as a compendium of simple, readily applicable remedies for the rapid treatment of patients. The extensive circulation and continued use of the *Euporiston* among late antique and medieval physicians is attested precisely by the numerous later interpolations attributed to the so-called Pseudo-Theodorus. In this sense, texts and interpolations of this kind contributed to the persistence and perceived reliability of remedies based on graphophagy.

A further example of the circulation of such prescriptions in Roman North Africa is provided by the anonymous *Antidotarium Bruxellense*. This medical treatise, likewise connected with the manuscript tradition of Theodorus Priscianus, dates to the sixth century. It attributed therapeutic efficacy against fever and against ailments of all kinds, both internal and external, to a series of mysterious names. These were to be written in ink on a clean sheet of paper, dissolved twice in three cups of hot water, and then administered to the patient.[67] No information is given concerning the composition of the ink, although the symbolic significance of the numerical sequence is noteworthy. As will become apparent, fever was frequently among the primary targets of graphophagic remedies.

Northern Africa constituted a particularly a favourable cultural environment for the application and circulation of such techniques. This may help

64 Britta K. Ager, *The Scent of Ancient Magic* (University of Michigan Press, 2022). On the medicinal properties of bay leaves, see Keith Singletary, "Bay Leaf: Potential Health Benefits," *Nutrition Today* 56, no. 4 (2021): 202–8.

65 Pseudo-Theodorus Priscianus, *Additamenta*, 308: "Item scribes intra calicem nomina infra scripta 'Dormiat ille Gaius Seius somnum humanum. KCЄ MIYYCaCB CON.' dices in calice et dabis ei cui voles, et statim."

66 Ibidem: "… ei dormiat ille quem peperit illa et ad nasum sibi teneat et olfaciat."

67 Ibid., 368.

to explain why significant parallels are found in the *Greek Magical Papyri*, a corpus of texts from Graeco-Roman Egypt roughly dating from the 2nd century BCE to the 5th century CE. The papyri contain spells, formulae, hymns, and detailed ritual instructions. As such, the collection is highly heterogeneous and reflects a wide spectrum of religious traditions and cultural practices. Whilst the label "magical" has been attributed by modern scholarship, the term also appears self-referentially within some of the texts themselves. Hans Betz considers them a collection of rituals and spells reflecting the content of underground magical books which were burned during the Roman imperial period and in late antiquity. More recently, David Frankfurter has suggested that such ritual practices were likely connected with third-to-fourth-century Egyptian priesthood.[68]

The cultural assumptions underlying the papyri take for granted the efficacy of the written word, including its therapeutic potential, and the idea that such power could be activated through physical contact. A remedy for a scorpion's sting, for example, prescribes the use of a piece of papyrus inscribed with mysterious characters, which was to be wrapped around the wound.[69] Pliny may well have regarded remedies of this kind eccentric or even nonsensical, yet his very inclusion of them reveals their cultural currency. In the *Historia naturalis*, when discussing the widespread use of language and chants for protection, he recalls an episode from Book XIX of the *Odyssey*, in which the sons of Autolycus heal a wound in Odysseus' thigh by binding it while reciting a *carmen* that successfully stanches the bleeding.[70] Was Pliny's citation of this Homeric precedent a way to legitimise a practice he personally doubted? His further claim that even Cato and Caesar trusted in charms seems to serve a similar rhetorical purpose.

---

68 *The Greek Magical Papyri in Translation Including the Demotic Spells*, ed. Hans Dieter Betz (The University of Chicago Press, 1986), xli; David Frankfurter, "Ritual Expertise in Roman Egypt and the Problem of the Category 'Magician,'" in *Envisioning Magic: A Princeton Seminar and Symposium*, ed. Peter Schäfer and Hans G. Kippenberg (Brill, 1997), 115–35.

69 PGM VII. 193–196.

70 Pliny the Elder, *Naturalis Historia*, xxviii.4.19–21: "Defigi quidem diris precationibus nemo non metuit. [...] Iam parietes incendiorum deprecationibus conscribuntur. neque est facile dictu, externa verba atque ineffabilia abrogent fidem validius an Latina et inopinata, quae inridicula videri cogit animus semper aliquid inmensum exspectans ac dignum deo movendo, immo vero quod numini imperet. Dixit Homerus profluvium sanguinis vulnerato femine Ulixen inhibuisse carmine, Theophrastus ischiadicos sanari, Cato prodidit luxatis membris carmen auxiliare, M. Varro podagris. Caesarem dictatorem post unum ancipitem vehiculi casum ferunt semper, ut primum consedisset, id quod plerosque nunc facere scimus, carmine ter repetito securitatem itinerum aucupari solitum."

Despite his own reservations, therefore, such practices had long enjoyed – and would continue to enjoy – considerable popularity in the Roman world, well into late antiquity, sustained by this double register of scepticism and practice. Much like the *Cyranides* – a Greek text of natural magic cataloguing the powers of stones, plants, and animals which circulated in a fluid form for centuries before being assembled around the fourth century and translated into Latin in 1169[71] – these practices assume that "essence and noun are perceived as identical."[72] These are just a few of several examples, rooted in ancient tradition, of what may be described as verbal homeopathy.[73]

Each text within the *corpus* of the Greek Magical Papyri simultaneously presents three essential components: the *praxeis* (πράξεις), that is, the actions to be performed; the *logoi* (λόγοι), namely the formulae to be written or spoken; and a material element, encompassing the substances required to carry out the ritual. This tripartite structure is exemplified by a memory spell that prescribes the use of a hieratic papyrus – upon which specific names are to be inscribed – together with a special ink.[74] This particularly valuable type of priestly papyrus (*hieratikē papyros*, ἱερατικὴ πάπυρος), produced from the central strips of the papyrus plant, was traditionally reserved for religious texts, as noted by Pliny.[75] Within the same *corpus* it is employed in a variety of contexts, most often for therapeutic, divinatory, and erotic purposes, as well as in curses.[76]

The names were to be written using the myrrh ink of Hermes. This ink was made from four drams of myrrh troglitis, three karian figs, seven pits of Nikolaus dates, seven dried pinecones, seven piths of single-stemmed wormwood, seven wings of the Hermaic ibis, and spring water;[77] the ingredients were to be burned together. Myrrh is an incense frequently mentioned in the

71 Christopher A. Faraone, *Ancient Greek Love Magic* (Harvard University Press, 1999), 121.

72 Monika Amsler, "*Voces Magicae* and Imperial/Late-Antique World-Making. Part 1," *ASDIWAL. Revue genevoise d'anthropologie et d'histoire des religions* 16 (2021): 29–43, at 38.

73 Eugene S. McCartney, "Verbal Homeopathy and the Etymological Story," *The American Journal of Philology* 48, no. 4 (1927): 326–30.

74 PGM I. 232–247.

75 Pliny the Elder, *Naturalis Historia*, xiii.23.74: "Hieratica appellabatur antiquitus religiosis tantum voluminibus dicata …"

76 E.g., PGM II. 1–64; PGM IV. 2006–2125, 2359–2372, and 3125–3171; PGM V. 306–369, and 370–446; PGM VII. 411–416, 579–590, and 969–972; PGM XIc. 1–19; PGM XIII. 1–343; PGM XIXb. 4–18.

77 On the papyri ink, see Olivier Bonnerot, Eleni Chronopoulou, and Ira Rabin, "Instrumental Analysis of the Inks from the Magical Papyrus P. Berol. Inv. 5026 (PGM ii / GEMF 30)," *Zeitschrift für Papyrologie und Epigraphik* 224 (2022): 267–73; Miriam Blanco Cesteros, "Written in Blood? Decoding Some Red Inks of the Greek Magical Papyri," in *Traces of Ink. Experiences of Philology and Replication*, ed. Lucia Raggetti (Brill, 2021), 33–56.

papyri for a wide range of purposes, both beneficial and harmful. Its ritual use can be traced back to Pharaonic Egypt, where it is attested as a component of an ink employed in a ritual from the *Book of the Dead* during the Eighteenth Dynasty.[78]

In the present context, myrrh plays a key role in the preparation of an ink frequently used within this *corpus*. The recurrent use of myrrh in general may indicate that it was relatively accessible. According to Dioscorides, myrrh troglitis (τρωγλῖτις σμύρνα), also known as troglodytis (τρωγλοδύτις), was the most expensive and most potent variety available, imported from Ethiopia.[79] The remaining ingredients are commonly prescribed in the papyri for the manufacture of inks, with the notable exception of the ibis wings, an animal sacred to Hermes Thoth, who was traditionally depicted with the head of an ibis and shown in the act of writing. Odd numbers had long been regarded as the most powerful, Virgil going as far as to say that they were the gods' favourites.[80]

The names to be written were the following:

> KAMBRĒ CHAMBRE SIXIŌPHI HARPON CHNOUPHI BRINTATĒNŌPHRIBRISKYLMA ARAOUAZAR BAMESEN KRIPHI NIPTOUMI CHMOUMAŌPH AKTIŌPHI ARTŌSE BIBIOU / BIBIOU SPHĒ SPHĒ NOUSI NOUSI SIEGŌ NOUCHA NOUCHA LINOUCHA LINOUCHA CHYCHBA CHYCHBA KAXIŌ CHYCHBA DĒTOPHŌTH II AA OO YY ĒĒ EE ŌŌ

They were then washed off into spring water drawn from seven different springs and were to be drunk on an empty stomach for seven days, while the moon was in the east. In this and in other similar cases, the ink differs from that used for writings not intended to be licked or ingested, such as texts written in gold or

78 Renata-Gabriela Tatomir, "To Cause 'To Make Divine' Through Smoke: Ancient Egyptian Incense and Perfume. An Inter- and Transdisciplinary Re-Evaluation of Aromatic Biotic Materials Used by the Ancient Egyptians," in *Moesica et Christiana – Studies in honor of Professor Alexandru Barnea*, ed. Adriana Panaite, Romeo Cîrjan, and Carol Căpiţă (Muzeul Brăilei "Carol I", Editura Istros, 2016), 665–78. Myrrh remained part of the Egyptian ritual tradition after the Arab conquest as one the key ingredients of "Egyptian ink," attributed to al-Qalalūsī in the seventh century. See Armin Schopen, *Tinten und Tuschen des arabisch-islamischen Mittelalters. Dokumentation – Analyse – Rekonstruktion* (Vandenhoeck & Ruprecht, 2006).

79 Pedanius Dioscorides of Anazarbus, *De materia medica*, trans. Lily Y. Beck (Olms-Weidmann, 2005), I.64.

80 Pliny the Elder, *Naturalis Historia*, xxviii.5.23: "cur inpares numeros ad omnia vehementiores credimus, idque in febribus dierum observatione intellegitur?"; Virgil, *Ecl.*, viii.75. See Tessa Morrison, "The Art of Early Medieval Number Symbolism," *Journal of the Australian Early Medieval Association* 2 (2006): 169–81.

silver inks.[81] As Fritz Graf has observed, such examples indicate that written material here functions not as communication but as ritual substance to be destroyed, ingested, and assimilated.[82] Unlike texts in libraries, where preservation equals value, these graphophagic texts achieve their purpose through erasure. When divine names are dissolved and drunk, the practitioner enacts a form of incorporative theology: the power of the deity enters the body not metaphorically but materially; the ink itself becomes a vector of sacred presence.

As this book aims to demonstrate, special words could transform food into a writing surface and, conversely, render different types of writing surfaces potentially edible. Understanding or comprehension was not required, since the practice did not constitute a form of person-to-person communication, but rather an interaction between the human and the (super)natural realm. At times, the very unintelligibility of names and formulae may have enhanced their authority and perceived efficacy, and the possibility that the scribes themselves were unaware of their meaning cannot be ruled out. Similar formulae may have been passed down over many generations, and even if knowledge of their original sense was lost, this did not diminish their presumed inner supernatural power.

Other instances attesting to the powers of graphophagy are found throughout the Greek Magical Papyri, where the ingestion or erasure of writing forms part of a coherent ritual logic rather than a series of isolated curiosities.[83] Across this heterogeneous corpus, four interrelated assumptions recur. First, writing operates within a material semiotics in which letters and names are treated as substances endowed with efficacy. Second, inscription is often completed through erasure: texts are written to be dissolved, licked away, or otherwise destroyed. Third, ritual efficacy is activated through sensorial engagement – taste, touch, and bodily incorporation – rather than through semantic comprehension. Finally, graphophagic practices rely on sympathetic correspondences linking natural materials, celestial bodies, divine powers, and the desired outcome of the rite.

Within this framework, a first group of rituals connects graphophagy to memory and cognition. One recipe intended to strengthen memory prescribes writing an Egyptian apotropaic symbol on a cinquefoil leaf using myrrh ink

81 Amsler, "*Voces Magicae* and Imperial/Late-Antique World-Making," 39, fn. 76.

82 Fritz Graf, "Magie et écriture : quelques réflexions," in *Écrire la magie dans l'antiquité : Actes du colloque international (Liège, 13–15 octobre 2011)* (Presses Universitaires de Liège, 2015), 227–38. See also PGM III. 410–23.

83 On these, see also *Handwörterbuch des deutschen Aberglaubens*. Vol. 8: *Silber–Vulkan*, ed. Hanns Bächtold-Stäubli and Eduard Hoffmann-Krayer (de Gruyter, 1937), 1156–7.

and keeping it in the mouth while sleeping.[84] The choice of cinquefoil is significant: its leaves are notably bitter owing to their high tannin content, and the ingestion of recognisable botanical substances may have created the sensory impression that some effect had indeed taken place – a kind of sensory validation of ritual efficacy.[85] The bitterness itself becomes evidence of the remedy's potency, transforming an unpleasant taste into a therapeutic sign.

A similar logic underlies a ritual in which an eight-letter mysterious name (I EE OO IAI) was written on a persea leaf (*Mimusops schimperi*), a tree regarded as sacred in ancient Egypt and associated with the sun, using a special ink made from the juice of the herb *kentritis*, honey, and myrrh. The name was to be licked every morning while facing the rising sun to secure the protection of the solar deity[86] – a procedure that, repeated daily, transforms ingestion into a sustained devotional practice rather than a one-time cure. In such cases, cognitive enhancement or protection is not achieved through reading or memorisation, but through the bodily assimilation of written signs embedded in a network of solar sympathetic associations.

A second cluster of examples places graphophagy within practices of mediation between humans and non-human agents, including the dead, animals, and supernatural entities. Contact with the deceased, for instance, could be established by placing in a corpse's mouth a flax leaf inscribed with the words "AZĒL BALEMACHŌ" in a special ink made from red ochre, burnt myrrh, fresh wormwood juice, evergreen, and flax.[87] Flax leaves recur in necromantic contexts, particularly in rituals aimed at interrogating corpses or skulls, and their use here underscores the role of writing as a material mediator rather than a communicative device.[88] Similar logics govern rites involving animal bodies, which function as liminal substrates through which dreams could be induced or erotic attraction compelled.[89] Within these contexts, graphophagy does not facilitate communication between human interlocutors, but rather

84 PGM II. 1–64.

85 Alan Sumler, "Ingesting Magic: Ingredients and Ecstatic Outcomes in the *Greek* and *Demotic Magical Papyri*," *Arion: A Journal of Humanities and the Classics* 25, no. 1 (2017): 99–126, at 121.

86 PGM IV. 475–829, 779–791. On the persea tree, see Stefano G. Caneva, "The Persea Tree from Alexander to Late Antiquity: A Contribution to the Cultural and Social History of Greco-Roman Egypt," *Ancient Society* 46 (2016): 39–66, esp. 40ff.

87 PGM IV. 2140–2144.

88 Christopher A. Faraone, "Necromancy Goes Underground: The Disguise of Skull- and Corpse-Divination in the Paris Magical Papyri (*PGM* IV 1928–2144)," in *Mantikê. Studies in Ancient Divination*, ed. Sarah Iles Johnston and Peter T. Struck (Brill, 2005), 255–82.

89 PGM XII, 107–21, 107–109; PGM XXXVI. 361–71. See also PDM Suppl. 101–116 and 117–130.

enables interaction with invisible or non-human powers by materially embedding written elements within organic bodies.

A third set of practices foregrounds the controlled destruction of writing as the locus of ritual efficacy. Licking, in particular, emerges as a liminal technique that occupies an intermediate position between reading, tasting, and swallowing.[90] Unlike full ingestion, licking allows for repeated contact and gradual erasure, maintaining ritual control over the written sign while still incorporating it bodily. One ritual prescribes writing a sacred stele text on both faces of a natron plaque:[91] one side was licked away, while wine or milk was poured over the other, collecting the dissolved ink inside a bowl to be drunk after a prescribed invocation.[92] Similarly, fear and anger could be subdued by writing a sign on a laurel leaf, holding it up to the sun, reciting a prayer to the god addressed as IAŌ OYŌ IŌ AIŌ OYŌ, and then licking the leaf clean.[93] In such cases, writing achieves its ritual purpose not by enduring, but by being materially transformed and eliminated.[94]

Across these examples,[95] writing grants material presence to ritual forces and to facilitate their assimilation through the body. Taken together, these practices show that graphophagy in the Greek Magical Papyri was not a marginal curiosity, but a coherent ritual logic grounded in: material semiotics (writing operates as a substance, not only as a carrier of meaning); tactility and bodily incorporation; sympathetic correspondences; and the performative destruction of writing as a means of engaging the (super)natural realm. Since perhaps comprehension was not always required, writing did not mediate between humans, but between matter and power.

There can be little doubt, therefore, that writing was intimately connected with multiple forms of power within the scribal cultures of Egypt, Judaism, and the Greek world. Writing transcended its role as a pragmatic technology; it was perceived as a means to imbue various objects – stone, wood, papyrus, food, and drink – with potent names and formulae, allowing it to act upon

90 Robert K. Ritner, *The Mechanics of Ancient Egyptian Magical Practice* (The Oriental Institute of the University of Chicago, 1993), 92–110. See also Id., "Horus on the Crocodiles: A Juncture of Religion and Magic in Late Dynastic Egypt," in *Religion and Philosophy in Ancient Egypt*, ed. William K. Simpson (Yale University Press, 1989), 103–16, esp. 106–8.

91 Natron is a mineral salt consisting of hydrated sodium carbonate.

92 PGM XIII. 1–343, 131–135. See also the parallels in PGM XIII. 343–646 and 646–734.

93 PGM XIII. 734–1077, 1043–1051.

94 Licking could also involve eggs as writing surfaces: PGM VII.505–528. Eggs held a distinctive place in the ritual practices attested in the papyri, particularly those of crows, falcons, and insects such as beetles and scarabs – the latter being regarded as apotropaic amulets and as symbols of rebirth and renewal.

95 See also PGM IV. 1716–1870, 1741–1745.

reality itself. Texts – much like images – were transmitted contagiously: they were conceived as physical and material media through which the power of words, names, and formulae could be conveyed into the human body.[96] This should not be surprising. Experimental studies have shown that, even in contemporary Western world, names and images are perceived as vectors of an entity's nature and quality, owing to associative modes of thought – that is, the assumption that "like attracts like," which lies at the core of Frazer's classical formulation of *sympathetic magic*.[97]

Graeco-Egyptian and Coptic papyri show that, in the early centuries of Christianity, a wide range of magical books and rolls circulated throughout the eastern Mediterranean among Jews, pagans, and Christians alike. The early Church appears to have been deeply concerned by their dissemination, to the point of mounting repeated campaigns aimed at prohibiting and destroying grimoires and other forms of occult literature.[98] By the time Christianity had spread into the western provinces, the idea that powers and qualities could be transferred contagiously from one object to another – as well as the belief in the generative efficacy of language – had long been well established.[99] For to think that "like produces like" is to think analogically, a mode of reasoning that nineteenth-century cultural evolutionists tended to characterise as a rudimentary way of understanding nature.

However, such practices were neither perceived as naïve by those who employed, taught, and transmitted them, nor were they grounded in elementary ideas and confined to cultures that would have been regarded as "primitive" even by late nineteenth-century standards. Quite the contrary. For the vast majority of human history prior to the scientific revolution, what are now labelled "science" and "magic" frequently coexisted and intersected without any clear sense of incompatibility.

96 Frankfurter, "The Magic of Writing in Mediterranean Antiquity," 635.

97 Paul Rozin, Linda Millman, and Carl Nemeroff, "Operation of the Laws of Sympathetic Magic in Disgust and Other Domains," *Journal of Personality and Social Psychology* 50, no. 4 (1986): 703–12; Id., Maureen Markwith, and Bonnie Ross, "The Sympathetic Magical Law of Similarity, Nominal Realism, and Neglect of Negatives in Response to Negative Labels," *Psychological Science* 1, no. 6 (1990): 383–84. Cf. James G. Frazer, *The Golden Bough: A Study in Magic and Religion*, abridged ed. (Macmillan, 1922), 11–48.

98 Gideon Bohak, "The Diffusion of the Greco-Egyptian Magical Tradition in Late Antiquity," in *Greco-Egyptian Interactions. Literature, Translation, and Culture, 500 BCE–300 CE*, ed. Ian Rutherford (Oxford University Press, 2016), 357–81; Frankfurter, "The Magic of Writing in Mediterranean Antiquity."

99 Jeremy Schott, "Language," in *Late Ancient Knowing: Explorations in Intellectual History*, ed. Catherine M. Chin and Moulie Vidas (University of California Press, 2015), 58–79.

Claiming that the power attributed to specific words or phrases can be absorbed by washing them from a writing surface underscores the belief in sympathetic connections – a foundational concept that permeated various ancient cultures, linking linguistic forms directly to their material effects. The term "sympathy" derives from the Greek *sympatheia* (συμπάθεια), formed of συν ("with, together") and πάθος ("feeling, emotion", "suffering"). It may be translated as "feeling together", or "suffering together," and was commonly rendered in Latin as *compassio*.[100] Belief in a sympathetic cosmos entailed a vision of reality in which: everything was potentially connected to everything else; sympathy and antipathy accounted for causal relationships between things; such connections were invisible to the human eye; action at a distance operated according to the same laws and occurred instantaneously; and, finally, the universe was conceived as a living organism. Moreover, the fact that the term *sympathy* derives from Greek reflects the centrality of this concept within Greek philosophical conceptualisations of nature.

A theory of "cosmic sympathy" can already be found in the writings of Posidonius of Apamea, a Stoic philosopher active between the second and the first century BCE.[101] While Aristotle and Plato had previously discussed sympathy, they tended to restrict its effects to relatively minor phenomena, such as the urge to urinate when near water, shivering in response to unpleasant sounds, or yawning when observing someone else yawn.[102] They understood sympathy as operating in specific instances of "co-affection." With Epicurus and, above all, the Stoics, however, sympathy was elevated to the status of a universal law. Plotinus, the founder of Neoplatonism, would later propose it as the very theory of everything that explained the functioning of the universe itself.

Within such a sympathetic cosmos, magic (μαγεία or γοητεία) did not constitute a failed attempt to rationalise nature, but rather the core engine embedded in the structure of the universe.[103] For Plotinus, the cosmos resembled an immense musical instrument, in which charms and prayers emitted resonant frequencies capable of producing desired effects. As with any musical instrument, success depended on knowing the correct notes, chords, and harmonies to exploit the occult relations of sympathy and antipathy that animated the living universe. Stones, plants, bodily substances, natural elements, and

100 Eric Schliesser, "Introduction: On Sympathy," in *Sympathy. A History*, ed. Eric Schliesser (Oxford University Press, 2015), 3–14, at 3.

101 Maraschi, Similia similibus curantur, 39–41.

102 René Brouwer, "Stoic Sympathy," in *Sympathy. A History*, 15–35, at 16–18.

103 Plotino, *Enneadi*, ed. Giovanni Reale and Roberto Radice (Mondadori, 2008), IV.4.40, 535.

words – spoken or written – set these cosmic strings vibrating. Plotinian's magic is not manipulative but participative: the practitioner does not coerce nature but aligns with its inherent patterns, generating what appear as instantaneous actions at a distance within the score of nature.[104]

Alongside the official principle of classical medicine, *contraria contrariis curantur*, the complementary notion of *similia similibus curantur* thus thrived by virtue of its ancient and authoritative pedigree.[105] This conceptual framework is fundamental to understanding why sympathy in general, and graphophagy in particular, enjoyed a considerably positive valuation from late antiquity into the early medieval period.

Ancient and late-antique graphophagic remedies were often marked by a pronounced syncretism and cultural hybridity.[106] Ideas, techniques, words, as well as the dosage, form, and qualitative value of letters and formulae were handed down across centuries, precisely because they were understood to be "the result of continued reasoning of observed, learned, and derived facts."[107]

104 Wendy E. Helleman, "Plotinus and Magic," *The International Journal of the Platonic Tradition* 4 (2010): 114–46.

105 Maraschi, "Mangiare preghiere, bere incantesimi," 99–100.

106 Ljuba M. Bortolani, *Magical Hymns from Roman Egypt: A Study of Greek and Egyptian Traditions of Divinity* (Cambridge University Press, 2016), 1–56; Ra'anan Boustan and Joseph E. Sanzo, "Christian Magicians, Jewish Magic, and the Shared Magical Culture of Late Antiquity," *Harvard Theological Review* 110, no. 2 (2017): 217–40. On syncretism, see also David Frankfurter, "Syncretism and the Holy Man in Late Antique Egypt," *Journal of Early Christian Studies* 11 (2003): 339–85.

107 Amsler, "*Voces Magicae* and Imperial/Late-Antique World-Making," 43.

CHAPTER 2

Ireland and Britain: the Normalisation of Graphophagy

Magic and *sympatheia* thus intersect categories such as religion, philosophy, and science. Indeed, these concepts overlap with the latter domains so deeply and with such historical continuity that their analytical separation is often counterproductive. Within these intersecting contexts, words played a crucial role.

In predominantly oral societies, words tend to be attributed fixed characteristics and structures – such as rhythmically balanced expressions, fixed formulae, and dense patterning – that may be compared to the formal stability of written words in literate cultures.[1] However, written words themselves may also be invested with intrinsic sacred or supernatural powers, as occurred in many regions of the world. Moreover, over the course of history, literacy has often inherited such powers from orality; in these cases, it could be further reinforced by qualities attributed to writing surfaces, inks, oral formulae, and other material and performative elements. Just as oral societies believed spoken words to be capable of affecting reality, so too did literate societies ascribe similar efficacy to written words, regardless of whether the performer fully understood their semantic content.[2]

For these reasons, Ireland constitutes a particularly important point of departure for understanding the circulation of graphophagic remedies in the early medieval West. The conventional account, articulated differently by scholars like James F. Kenney and Richard Sharpe, holds that Irish Christianity synthesised Celtic and Roman elements while maintaining unusual openness to practices that elsewhere would have been condemned as pagan survivals.[3] Yet, it should not be assumed that "pagan" and "Christian" practices can be neatly distinguished, that the former survived into the latter through processes of accommodation or disguise. More likely, Irish Christians did not accommodate pagan practices into Christianity but rather operated within a Christian worldview that had never excluded certain forms of ritual action. In fact,

1 Ong, *Orality and Literacy*, 35.

2 Cardona, *Antropologia della scrittura*.

3 James F. Kenney, *The sources for the early history of Ireland: an introduction and guide* (Columbia University Press, 1929); Richard Sharpe, "Some Problems Concerning the Organization of the Church in Early Medieval Ireland," *Peritia* 3 (1984): 58–72.

 | HTTPS://DOI.ORG/10.1163/9789004765528-004

graphophagic remedies appear in monastic manuscripts not as embarrassing relics but as practical technologies fully compatible with Christian devotion.

Having played a major role in the Christianisation of Europe, Ireland acquired the reputation of a holy land – or even of a heaven on Earth.[4] It was portrayed as a land where rivers of milk and honey flowed,[5] endowed with a mild climate and an abundance of food,[6] all features conventionally associated with Edenic landscapes.[7]

This transformation of earlier perceptions was significant. Roman authors had traditionally depicted Ireland as a remote land inhabited by barbarous peoples and characterised by uncivilised customs. With Christianisation and the missionary activity of itinerant Irish monks across large parts of Europe, however, the island came to be reimagined as an Edenic space.[8] From a symbolic perspective, another feature assumed particular importance: the complete absence of snakes, a trait already noted by Isidore of Seville.[9] This motif, typical of hagiographic tradition, served to emphasise the connection between Irish saints and biblical prophets, while simultaneously reinforcing the idea of Ireland as an exceptionally holy land.[10] Legend aside, this peculiarity can be understood as a natural feature that was subsequently invested with religious meaning. The absence of snakes in Ireland does in fact correspond to ecological reality: for geological reasons, the island has no native species of snakes, much like other islands such as Iceland, Greenland and New Zealand.[11]

---

4 Dagmar Ó Riain-Raedel, "The Other Paradise: Perceptions of Ireland in the Middle Ages," in *Between the Islands and the Continent: Papers on Hiberno-Scandinavian-Continental Relations in the Early Middle Ages*, ed. Rudolf Simek and Asya Ivanova (Fassbaender, 2013), 167–92.

5 As in Ex 3:17.

6 *Bede's ecclesiastical history of the English people*, ed. and trans. Beltram Colgrave and R.A.B. Mynors (Clarendon Press, 1969), I, 1, 18.

7 Massimo Montanari, *Il cibo come cultura* (Laterza, 2006).

8 See for example *L'Irlanda e gli irlandesi nell'alto medioevo*. Atti della LVII Settimana di Studio (Spoleto 16–21 2009) (CISAM, 2010).

9 Isidoro di Siviglia, *Etimologie o origini*, II, 14.6.

10 Alexander H. Krappe, "St. Patrick and the Snakes," *Traditio* 5 (1947): 323–30. On the hagiographic model, see Jennifer O'Reilly, *History, Hagiography and Biblical Exegesis. Essays on Bede, Adomnán and Thomas Becket* (Routledge, 2019); Andrea Maraschi, "I miracoli alimentari di San Colombano: l'originalità, la tradizione e la simbologia," *Studi Medievali* 52 (2011): 517–76. On St. Patrick and snakes, see Gerald of Wales, *Topographia Hibernica*, in Id., *Opera*, 8 vols., vol. 5, ed. James F. Dimock (Longmans, Green, Reader, and Dyer, 1867), d. I, ch. 28, 62.

11 Anthony J. Stuart, "Insularity and Quaternary Vertebrate Faunas in Britain and Ireland," in *Island Britain: A Quaternary Perspective*, ed. Richard C. Preece (Geological Society of

Bede addresses the evil symbolism of the snake at length in his commentaries on the Book of Genesis, where he discusses the serpent as the enemy of all animals, a physical embodiment of death, and a symbolic representation of temptation and attachment to earthly desires. Because snakes crawl rather than stand upright like humans, they are unable to look upwards towards the heavens, a posture that, for Bede, further underscores their association with the terrestrial and the sinful.[12]

In the *Historia ecclesiastica*, completed in 731, Bede places particular emphasis on the material, rather than purely meta-physical, reality of *serpentes*. Most interestingly, he mentions empirical attempts to test whether snakes could actually survive in Ireland, describing how they were imported by sea from Britannia in order to observe their fate upon reaching the island:

> No reptile is ever seen there, and no serpent can survive. For serpents often brought there from Britain perish as soon as the ship approaches the land and they are touched by the air's scent. Rather, almost everything originating from that island possesses properties that counteract venom. Indeed, we have seen some individuals bitten by a serpent be cured: after scraping the leaves of books brought from Ireland and putting the scrapings into water to drink, they experienced the venom's whole strength vanish and the swelling of the body subside entirely.[13]

This passage reveals Bede's remarkable integration of sympathetic theory into Christian natural philosophy. The antidote – manuscript shavings mixed with water – operates through transferred sacred virtue: the material substrate of Irish books, produced in a holy land, acquires antivenomous properties.

Bede presents empirical testimony to authenticate a practice grounded in sympathetic logic: the concept of *sympatheia* did not originate within a Judeo-Christian intellectual framework, yet Bede presents it as compatible

London, 1995), 111–25; J. Alan Holman, *Pleistocene Amphibians and Reptiles in Britain and Europe* (Oxford University Press, 1998), 207–8.

12 Venerable Bede, *Libri quatuor in principium Genesis usque ad nativitatem Isaac et eiectionem Ismahelis adnotationum*, ed. Charles W. Jones, CCSL 118A (Brepols, 1967).

13 *Bede's ecclesiastical history*, I, 1, 18: "nullum ibi reptile uideri soleat, nullus uiuere serpens ualeat; nam saepe illo de Brittania adlati serpentes, mox ut, proximante terris nauigio, odore aeris illius adtacti fuerint, intereunt; quin potius omnia pene, quae de eadem insula sunt, contra uenenum ualent. Denique uidimus, quibusdam a serpente percussis, rasa folia codicum, qui de Hibernia fuerant, et ipsam rasuram aquae inmissam ac potui datam, talibus protinus totam uim ueneni grassantis, totum inflati corporis absumsisse ac sedasse tumorem."

with Christian cosmology. This is, to some extent, understandable, since the biblical tradition itself includes notable precedents. One such example is the bronze serpent built by Moses at the Lord's command to save the Israelites from the creature's venom: like cures like, at least when sanctioned by God's will.[14]

While biblical precedents do exist, the practice of making healing potions by mixing parchment scrapings endowed with special virtues can hardly be described as a standard Judeo-Christian ritual. Yet, in Bede's writings the concepts of συμπάθεια and αντιπάθεια – concepts originally rooted in pre-Christian religious and philosophical traditions – emerge as fully integrated within a Christian framework.

A little further south, other Christian communities prepared similar mixtures by scraping dust from the tombs of saints – for instance, at Tours, from the grave of St. Martin.[15] This suggests that Christian mentalities shared the idea that miraculous healing powers invested in objects could be absorbed through ingestion, even though this does not imply that written formulae were regarded as equivalent to holy relics. It may be noted that the efficacy of Irish potions stemmed from the content of the manuscripts themselves, most likely religious texts. Bede's account, however, seems to suggest that the very material of the codices, by having been produced in a holy land, was itself imbued with a potency inimical to evil.[16]

Putting God's will to the test was not a typical Christian attitude.[17] And yet, the antipathy of serpents towards Ireland became the object of what were presented as actual experiments. According to Bede, several attempts were made

14 Num 21:6–9. See also Ex 7:8–12.

15 Maraschi, Similia similibus curantur, 67–84. For later Irish parallels, see Deborah Hayden, "From the 'King of the Waters' to Curative Manuscripts: Water and Medicine in Medieval Irish Textual Culture," in *The Elements in the Medieval World: Interdisciplinary Perspectives. Water*, ed. Marilina Cesario, Hugh Magennis, and Elisa Ramazzina (Brill, 2024), 75–98, at 86–7. See also Charles Freeman, *Holy Bones, Holy Dust: How Relics Shaped the History of Medieval Europe* (Yale University Press, 2011); Stephen Wilson "Introduction," in Id., *Saints and their Cults. Studies in Religious Sociology, Folklore and History* (Cambridge University Press, 1983), 1–54, at 19–20.

16 It should be noted that serpents, like worms, represented embodiments of different types of disease in Anglo-Saxon and Scandinavian medical traditions. In early English medical remedies, ailments caused by snakes or worms are cured by means of formulae containing Irish linguistic forms. Hayden, "From the 'King of the Waters' to Curative Manuscripts," 77; Ciaran Arthur, *"Charms," Liturgies, and Secret Rites in Early Medieval England* (Boydell&Brewer, 2018), 73–80.

17 On the Frazerian distinction between coercion and invocation with regards to "magic" and religion, see: Fritz Graf, "Prayer in Magic and Religious Ritual," in *Magika Hiera: Ancient Greek Magic and Religion*, ed. Christopher A. Faraone and Dirk Obbink (Oxford

to introduce snakes from Britannia to Ireland, but the animals died before even reaching land, as soon as they inhaled its saintly air. In this respect, Bede is clearly reworking his sources – Solinus[18] and Isidore – who mention the absence of snakes in Ireland, the lack of certain birds, and, more generally, the land's relations of antipathy, including those involving bees. Between hagiographic *topoi* and matters of faith, Bede's account plausibly reflects widespread mental attitudes and suggests that early medieval religious thought continued to harbour, whether consciously or not, the operative categories of pre-Christian ritual thinking.[19]

The material reality attributed to written words can be inferred from a text preserved in the Exeter Book, a manuscript dating to the second half of the tenth century that contains both secular and religious works, including a collection of riddles.[20] Riddle no. 47 is particularly relevant to any discussion of the ingestion and destruction of writing. This brief six-line poem, adapted from a Latin model attributed to Symphosius,[21] describes a scene that must have been familiar in monastic *scriptoria*: a moth or bookworm gnawing its way through a manuscript leaf.[22]

Both the Latin and the Old English version emphasise that the creature does not know what letters are. Although it may consume an entire book, it acquires no knowledge and becomes no wiser for having done so. The *enigma* thus contrasts two modes of contact with writing. On the one hand, the animal devours text purely driven by survival instinct rather than understanding. On the other hand, the human reader engages with written words as repositories of meaning and knowledge. Yet, this contrast presupposes a crucial shared premise: written words, unlike oral ones, are materially embedded in the manuscript leaf and are therefore susceptible to physical destruction.

University Press, 1991), 188–97; Karen L. Jolly, "Medieval Magic: Definitions, Beliefs, Practices," in *Witchcraft and Magic in Europe: 3. The Middle Ages*, 1–72, at 6.

18 Caius Julius Solinus, *Collectanea Rerum Memorabilium*, ed. Theodor Mommsen (Weidmann, 1895), 22, 2.3, 112.

19 Arthur, *"Charms," Liturgies, and Secret Rites.*

20 Exeter, Cathedral Library 3501. Edited version in: Richard Marsden, *The Cambridge Old English Reader* (Cambridge University Press, 2004).

21 It has been suggested that the Latin text may have been composed in the late fourth or the early fifth century. Erin Sebo, "*In scirpo nodum*: Symphosius' Reworking of the Riddle Form," in *The Muse at Play: Riddles and Wordplay in Greek and Latin Poetry*, ed. Jan Kwapzt, David Petrain, and Mikolaj Szymanski (de Gruyter, 2013), 184–95, at 184.

22 Marsden, *The Cambridge Old English Reader*, 316. I wish to thank Hugh Magennis for bringing this example to my attention.

The riddle makes this point explicitly by characterising the worm as a *thief in the dark* who *steals* words from the folio.[23] Letters and texts are imagined as tangible entities that can be eaten, lost, or erased. What distinguishes the worm from the human, however, is not the act of ingestion itself, but its efficacy. When consumed by an animal, writing is reduced to nourishment and annihilated; when consumed – literally or metaphorically – by a human, it can transmit knowledge, power, or efficacy precisely because it is conceived as a codified material thing. In this sense, the riddle offers a striking negative counterpart to graphophagic practices: it confirms that the ingestion of writing was imaginable and intelligible within early medieval culture, while simultaneously insisting that meaning and potency depended not merely on consumption, but on the culturally sanctioned conditions under which written words were destroyed, assimilated, and made operative.

This artfully crafted metaphorical logic is echoed from another angle in Bede's *Historia ecclesiastica*, specifically in Book IV, which recounts the story of the herdsman Cædmon and his miraculous acquisition of poetic skill.[24] According to the account, Cædmon, an elderly lay brother at the monastery of Whitby, was unable to sing and therefore habitually left communal feasts before any singing began. One night, after departing from such a gathering, he falls asleep and is visited in a dream by an unknown figure who commands him to sing. Initially reluctant, Cædmon is pressed to comply, and he is instructed to sing on the theme of *principium creaturarum* – "the beginning of created things."

As a result, Cædmon begins to sing, spontaneously composing the now-famous *Hymn*, the oldest surviving in Old English, dating from the second half of the seventh century.[25] Both the gift of poetic composition and the content itself are divinely granted,[26] a mechanism closely analogous to hagiographical narratives describing how sixth-century hymnographer Romanos Melodos acquired the ability to compose sacred hymns.[27] In both cases, inspiration or knowledge is mediated externally and transmitted directly into the recipient,

23 Hugh Magennis, *The Cambridge Introduction to Anglo-Saxon Literature* (Cambridge University Press, 2011), 73–75.

24 On this story, see Daniel P. O'Donnell, *Cædmon's Hymn: A multimedia study, archive and edition* (D.S. Brewer, SEENET, and The Medieval Academy, 2005).

25 Edited in Elliott Van Kirk Dobbie, ed. *The Anglo-Saxon Minor Poems* (Columbia University Press, 1942), 105–6.

26 Ruth Wehlau, "Rumination and Re-Creation: Poetic Instruction in *The Order of the World*," *Florilegium* 13 (1994): 65–77, at 66.

27 Sean W. Anthony, *Muhammad and the Empires of Faith: The Making of the Prophet of Islam* (University of California Press, 2020), 219–20. More on this later.

bypassing ordinary learning, a motif that resonates with the material and performative logic of graphophagic and other ritual practices: power, meaning, or skill can be transmitted by extraordinary channels, whether divine, material, or symbolic.

Bede presents this story as marking the official beginning of Christian poetry in Old English verse, itself a conscious Christian appropriation of a long-standing pre-literate and pre-Latinate poetic tradition.[28] Upon waking from the dream, Cædmon retains full memory of the experience and is brought before the abbess, to whom he describes his vision and sings his hymn. He is then assigned a test: he must translate a sacred text into verse, which he successfully completes overnight. Recognised as divinely gifted, Cædmon joins the abbey's religious community.

Thereafter, he is taught about "the whole course of sacred history," committing it to memory and ruminating over it, "like some clean animal chewing the cud"[29] – an allusion to the Hebrew distinctions of purity and impurity articulated in Leviticus 11 and Deuteronomy 14. This metaphor, which Bede also employs in his Easter vigil homily, evokes the monastic practice of listening to, internalising, and digesting.[30] It resonates closely with the logic of graphophagy: texts are materially present, ingested through reading or recitation, and transformed into knowledge and spiritual nourishment through deliberate, disciplined engagement.

Pronouncing the words of a text aloud, with one's lips moving in the act of reading, was thus likened to a form of mastication and spiritual nourishment. This metaphor must have carried particular force in a society that believed the powers inherent in words and symbols could be activated through their ingestion – a belief fully endorsed, at least from a Christian and hagiographical perspective.[31]

---

28 Andy Orchard, "The Word Made Flesh: Christianity and Oral Culture in Anglo-Saxon Verse," *Oral Tradition* 24, no. 2 (2009): 293–318, at 293.

29 *Bede's ecclesiastical history*, IV, xxiv, 416: "susceptumque in monasterium cum omnibus suis fratrum cohorti adsociauit, iussitque illum seriem sacrae historiae doceri. At ipse cuncta, quae audiendo discere poterat, rememorando secum et quasi mundum animal ruminando, in carmen dulcissimum conuertebat, suauiusque resonando doctores suos uicissim auditores sui faciebat."

30 Jean Leclercq, *The Love of Learning and the Desire for God. A Study of Monastic Culture* (Fordham University Press, 1974 [1961]), 89ff.; Philip J. West, "Rumination in Bede's Account of Cædmon," *Monastic Studies* 12 (1976): 217–26. The same metaphor is used by Quintilian (*Inst. orat.*, xi.ii.41), who compares meditation over a text and memorisation with the action of rechewing one's food.

31 Daniel Dubuisson, "Les talismans du roi Cormac et les trois functions," *Revue historique* 250, no. 508 (1973): 289–94, at 292; R.J.S. Barrett-Lennard, *Healing after the New Testament:*

Two fifteenth-century versions of the *Life of St. Columba*, preserved in the *Leabhar Breac*[32] and in the *Book of Lismore*,[33] contain a short passage that casts light on the intersection of Christian and pre-Christian ideas about graphophagy. Columba, otherwise known as Colm Cille (521–597), studied under Finnian of Clonard, one of the founding figures of Irish monasticism, and later established the renowned monastery of Iona in the Inner Hebrides, off Scotland's western coast.[34] Numerous sources recount his life, including works by Cumméne, abbot of Iona (657–669), his successor Adomnán (679–704), and Bede. Columba was of noble birth, the son of a king, and a member of the Uí Néill clan of Gartan.

The *Vita Sancti Columbae* preserved in the *Leabhar Breac* and the *Book of Lismore* bears little resemblance to the much earlier account by Adomnán. This version displays distinctive features, notably its homiletic structure – a characteristic shared with the lives of Patrick, Brigid, and Martin contained in the same *Leabhar Breac*. It remains unclear to what extent the author of this

---

Some Approaches to Healing in the Second, Third, and Fourth Centuries (University Press of America, 1994), 330.

32 The manuscript (RIA 23 P 16) dates to ca. 1408–11 and is preserved at the Royal Irish Academy in Dublin. It was compiled by a single scribe (possibly Murchadh Riabhach Ó Cuindlis) and includes religious texts in Latin and Irish. It was likely intended for a religious community or a churchman. See James F. Kenney, "Religious Literature and Ecclesiastical Culture," in Id., *The Sources for the Early History of Ireland: An Introduction and Guide. Volume 1: Ecclesiastical* (Octagon, 1966), 622–744, at 739; Tom ter Horst, *Codeswitching in the Irish-Latin* Leabhar Breac: *Mediæval Homiletic Culture* (Lot, 2017); Tomás Ó Concheanainn, "The Scribe of the Leabhar Breac," *Ériu* 24 (1973): 64–79, at 65. Facsimile edition: *Leabhar Breac, the Speckled Book, Otherwise Styled Leabhar M'or D'una Daighre, the Great Book of Dun Doighre; A Collection of Pieces in Irish and Latin, Compiled from Ancient Sources about the Close of the Fourteenth Century*, ed. Seosamh Ó Longáin and John J. Gilbert (Royal Irish Academy House, 1872–76).

33 The *Book of Lismore* was compiled in the fifteenth century by at least three scribes, one of whom being Aonghus Ó Callanáin. It might have been commissioned by Finghin Mac Carthaigh Riabach and his wife Caitlín. It was not intended for a monastic library anyways, but more likely for a lay beneficiary. The manuscript is preserved at the University College Cork, and includes hagiographic texts as well as works of different genres, such as Marco Polo's *Milione*: this reflects the interests of Gaelic and Anglo-Irish nobles of the time. Brian Ó Cuív, "Observations on the Book of Lismore," *Proceedings of the Royal Irish Academy. Section C: Archaeology, Celtic Studies, History, Linguistics, Literature* 83C (1983): 269–92; Donnchadh Ó Corráin, ed., Clavis Litterarum Hibernensium: *Medieval Irish Books & Texts* (*c. 400–c. 1600*) (Brepols, 2017); Caoimhín Breatnach, "Book of Lismore," in *Medieval Ireland. An Encyclopedia*, ed. Seán Duffy (Routledge, 2005), 279–80. The text can be found in: "Life of Colomb Cille," in *Lives of saints, from the Book of Lismore*, ed. Whitley Stokes (Clarendon, 1890), 168–81; Robert A.S. Macalister, ed., *The book of Mac Carthaigh Riabhach, otherwise the Book of Lismore* (The Stationery Office, 1950).

34 He also founded monasteries at Derry, Durrow, and Kells.

fifteenth-century hagiography drew upon earlier traditions or how much the text reflects the context of its own time. As Richard Sharpe has observed, "the writing of hagiography can hardly fail to reflect the milieu in which it is carried out."[35] This observation is particularly relevant here: even if the passage under analysis were a literary invention by the author that was later copied into the *Leabhar Breac* and the *Book of Lismore*,[36] it nevertheless provides valuable insights into the mindset of a fifteenth-century Irish Christian cleric. Whitley Stokes further notes that this version preserves certain "Irish superstitions,"[37] and that linguistic evidence suggests that the author did indeed draw upon older sources – a conclusion that applies equally to the *Book of Lismore*.[38]

The story of how Columba learned to read recalls Cædmon's, yet it emphasises the power of ingested letters. Most notably, it involves a druid. A distinctive feature of Irish hagiography is the coexistence of saints-to-be with members of the learned priestly class from pre-Christian Celtic society.[39] Druids were regarded as intermediaries between this world and the Otherworld, custodians of law and tradition, and wielders of significant social influence.

It is no wonder that a certain tension permeates the texts when druids encounter their new Christian counterparts:[40] "the demons of today could be the gods of yesterday or tomorrow," Jacqueline Borsje observes.[41] In this sense, druids functioned in Ireland much as μάγοι and *magi* did in classical and late antiquity – priests of an illicit religion, opposed to the true power of God.[42] Hagiographic narratives often depict druids as antagonists, ultimately defeated through the miracles of saints. Yet, despite these conflicts, druids and saints shared an important societal function: both served the community

35 Richard Sharpe, *Medieval Irish Saints' Lives. An Introduction to Vitae Sanctorum Hiberniae* (Clarendon, 1991), 35.

36 Since the two versions are equivalent, I will henceforth refer to the version preserved in the older of the two manuscripts, the *Leabhar Breac*.

37 *Three Middle-Irish Homilies on the Lives of Saints Patrick, Brigit and Columba*, ed. Whitley Stokes (privately printed, 1877), viii.

38 *Lives of saints, from the Book of Lismore*, xlv.

39 Andrea Maraschi and Francesca Tasca, *Food, Heresies, and Magical Boundaries in the Middle Ages* (Amsterdam University Press, 2024), 125–53.

40 Anne Ross, "Ritual and the Druids," in *The Celtic World*, ed. Miranda J. Green (Routledge, 1995), 423–44, at 423.

41 Jacqueline Borsje, "Druids, Deer and 'Words of Power:' Coming to Terms with Evil in Medieval Ireland," in *Coping with Evil in Religion and Culture. Case Studies*, ed. Nelly Van Doorn-harder and Lourens Minnema (Rodopi, 2008), 25–49, at 30.

42 Jacqueline Borsje, "Witchcraft and Magic," in *Medieval Ireland. An Encyclopedia*, 518–20. "Magic" was associated to other figures as well: Jacqueline Borsje and Fergus Kelly, "'The Evil Eye' in Early Irish Literature and Law," *Celtica* 24 (2003): 1–39.

through the exercise of their powers.[43] Indeed, the learned class of druids retained respect in Christian Ireland until the eighth century, even as the social and religious landscape began to change.[44] As a result, druids occupy a complex role in Irish hagiography, at times cast in opposition, but occasionally portrayed positively, reflecting both continuity and transformation in the use and perception of ritual knowledge.

In keeping with hagiographic conventions, the opening episodes of Columba's life foreshadows his extraordinary future – a pattern that holds true in Adomnán's account, too. Much like another prominent Irish saint, Columbanus, Columba's early life is marked by prophetic signs: for instance, a sphere of fire is seen above the sleeping child, signalling his status as a chosen intermediary between God and His people. Equally significant is Columba's education, which provides further indication of his bright fate:

> After his birth he was straightaway taken to be baptized by Cruithnechán, son of Cellachán, the noble priest, and he fostered him afterwards, being so bidden by an angel of God. Now, when came the time for him to read, the cleric went to a certain spaeman [*fáith*, which corresponds to Lat. *vatis*] who was biding in the country, to ask him when the boy ought to begin. When the spaeman had scanned the sky, he said, "Write for him his alphabet now." It was thereafter written on a cake [*bairgin*], and in this wise Colombcille ate the cake, to wit, half thereof to the east of the water and the other half to the west of the water. The spaeman said, through the gift of spaedom, "So shall the territory of this son be, to wit, half thereof to the east of the sea, that is in Scotland, and the other half to the west of the sea, that is in Ireland."[45]

The glory of the future saint was destined to shine on both lands. Columba quickly mastered the alphabet, but his talents extended beyond literacy: he also quickly acquired the gift of preaching. Not long after, during the Christmas celebrations, he accompanied the priest Cruithnechán to visit Brugach, Bishop of Raith Enaigh (Raymoghy). The bishop invited Cruithnechán to join him in

43 Ross, "Ritual and the Druids," 423.

44 Meanwhile, *vates* and bards – other learned figures of Celtic Ireland – were also slowly downgraded. Fergus Kelly, *A Guide to Early Irish Law* (Dublin Institute for Advanced Studies, 1988), 60; Barry Cunliffe, *Druids: A Very Short Introduction* (Oxford University Press, 2010), 95.

45 *Betha Colaim Chille. Life of Columcille. Compiled by Manus O'Donnell in 1532. Edited and translated from manuscript Rawlinson B. 514 in the Bodleian Library, Oxford*, ed. Andrew O'Kelleher and Gertrude Schoepperle (University of Illinois, 1918), 44–5; *On the Life of Saint Columba*, in *Three Middle-Irish Homilies*, 90–125, at 103.

leading the office, but the priest was so overcome with embarrassment at the thought of reciting the Hours alongside the bishop that he was unable to read the psalm *Misericordias Dei*. At that moment, Columba stepped forward without hesitation and sang the psalm in his place, despite having only just learned the alphabet. This remarkable feat was regarded as miraculous and marked the beginning of Columba's renown as one divinely chosen.

The priest Cruithnechán and the pagan soothsayer (*fáith*) represent learned authorities from two different religious systems, yet the Christian cleric seeks guidance from his pagan counterpart. The *fáith*, skilled in divination, interprets signs in the sky and answers Cruithnechán's question: Columba must learn to read at once. Notably, however, the soothsayer does not specify the method of instruction; it is Cruithnechán who picks a cake. From which the child will learn the alphabet by *eating*.

Stories of this sort were likely intended as idealised representations of the past,[46] suggesting a narrative of peaceful and productive transition from pagan to Christian authority.[47] If so, why a cake? Could it be a trivial narratological choice? The choice of a cake as the medium of learning strikes modern readers as odd, but dismissing it as hagiographic fancy misses what the episode reveals about Irish conceptions of pedagogy, materiality, and transformation. Ingesting the alphabet aligns with broader traditions of graphophagy and sympathetic assimilation: knowledge and power are transferred through literal consumption of letters, echoing motifs of spiritual and intellectual nourishment found elsewhere in early medieval literature. The cake thus serves as a culturally intelligible metaphor for a learned, transformative, and, above all, embodied pedagogy – one that would likely have been comprehensible to an Irish monastic audience steeped in both Latin learning and indigenous traditions of oral transmission.

Hagiography often conveyed stories with fantastic elements (i.e., miracles), yet the act of writing letters on the cake is not a miracle in itself. The practice of inscribing letters on food – including cakes – predates these accounts and is attested in Talmudic tradition.[48] Classical authors also reference analogous methods: Horace mentions letter-shaped pastries used to teach children the

46 John Carey, "The Three Rings Required of a Poet," *Ériu* 48 (1997): 41–58.

47 Katja Ritari, "From Pagan to Christian in the 7th century Irish Hagiography," *Studia Celtica Fennica* 1 (2004): 14–23.

48 Gérard Haddad, *Eating the Book: Dietary Rites and Paternal Function*, trans. David Jacobson (Agincourt Press, 2013), 91; Henri Gaidoz, "Les gâteaux alphabétiques," *Mélanges Rénier. Recuil de travaux publiés par l'École Pratique des Hautes Études* 73 (1887): 1–8.

alphabet,[49] while Quintilian, later echoed by St. Jerome, recommended letting children play with ivory letters as toys.[50]

Even though direct continuity of these educational practices is difficult to establish, material and iconographic evidence attest to their persistence. Abecedaries and inscribed boards appear among wealthy families in the late Middle Ages,[51] and archaeological finds include bowls similarly marked with the alphabet to aid in learning Latin,[52] helping children to associate written signs with specific sounds – a technique noted by the twelfth-century bishop John of Salisbury.[53] Edible alphabets, also documented in fifteenth-century Florence,[54] were all the more useful because children could associate a useful activity with a pleasant, consumable reward.[55] A northern Italian manuscript from the mid-fourteenth century (fig. 4) even personifies Grammar as a woman,

49 Quinto Orazio Flacco, *Le satire*, in Id., *Le opere*, ed. Tito Colamarino and Domenico Bo (UTET, 2013), I, i, 25: "Ut pueris olim dant crustula blandi / doctores, elementa velint ut discere prima".

50 Quintiliano, *L'istituzione oratoria*, ed. Rino Faranda and Piero Pecchiura (UTET, 2003), I, i, 26: "Non excludo autem, id quod est notum irritandae ad discendum infantiae gratia, eburneas etiam litterarum formas in lusum offerre, et si quid aliud, quo magis illa aetas gaudeat, inveniri potest, quod tractare, intueri, nominare iucundum est"; *Select letters of St. Jerome*, ed. F.A. Wright (Putnam, 1933), 107.4: "Fiant ei litterae vel buxeae vel eburneae et suis nominibus appellentur. Ludat in eis, ut et lusus eius eruditio sit".

51 Michael Clanchy, "Did Mothers Teach their Children to Read?," in *Motherhood, Religion, and Society in Medieval Europe, 400–1400. Essays Presented to Henrietta Leyser*, ed. Conrad Leyser and Lesley Smith (Routledge, 2011), 129–53, at 151; Robert D. Black, *Humanism and Education in Medieval and Renaissance Italy* (Cambridge University Press, 2001), 35–8; Danièle Alexandre-Bidon, "La lettre volée. Apprendre à lire à l'enfant au Moyen Âge," *Annales E.S.C.* 44 (1989): 953–92; Ead., "Abécédaires et alphabets éducatifs du XIIIe à la fin du XVe siècle," *Nouvelles de l'Estampe* 90 (1986): 6–10; Ead., *Alphabets: 1470–1700 : À lire, à dire, à écrire, à broder*, Catalogue de l'exposition (Paris, Bibliothèque Nationale, Réserve des Livres Rares et Precieux, 1990); *Tables Florentines. Écrire et manger avec Franco Sacchetti*, ed. Jacqueline Brunet and Odile Redon (Stock, 1984).

52 Suzanne Reynolds, *Medieval Reading: Grammar, Rhetoric and the Classical Text* (Cambridge University Press, 1996), 7–8.

53 John of Salisbury, *Metalogicon*, ed. John B. Hall and Katharine S.B. Keats-Rohan, CCCM 98 (Brepols, 1991), I, 13, 32: "… littere autem, id est figure, primum vocum indices sunt."

54 Matteo Palmieri, *Vita civile*, ed. Gino Belloni (Sansoni, 1982), 24; *Giovanni Rucellai ed il suo zibaldone. I: 'Il zibaldone quaresimale,'* ed. Alessandro Perosa (Warburg Institute, 1960), 14. See Christiane Klapisch-Zuber, "Le chiavi fiorentine di Barbablu: l'apprendimento della lettura a Firenze nel XV secolo," *Quaderni Storici* 57 (1984): 765–92, at 786; Robert D. Black, *Education and Society in Florentine Tuscany. Teachers, Pupils and Schools, c. 1250–1500* (Brill, 2007), 121–2.

55 Alexandre-Bidon, "La lettre volée," 971. For other ordinary uses of graphophagy (such as bread stamps), see Peter Kruschwitz, "Inhabiting a Lettered World: Exploring the Fringes of Roman Writing Habits," *Bulletin of the Institute of Classical Studies* 59, no. 1 (2016): 26–41, at. 29ff.

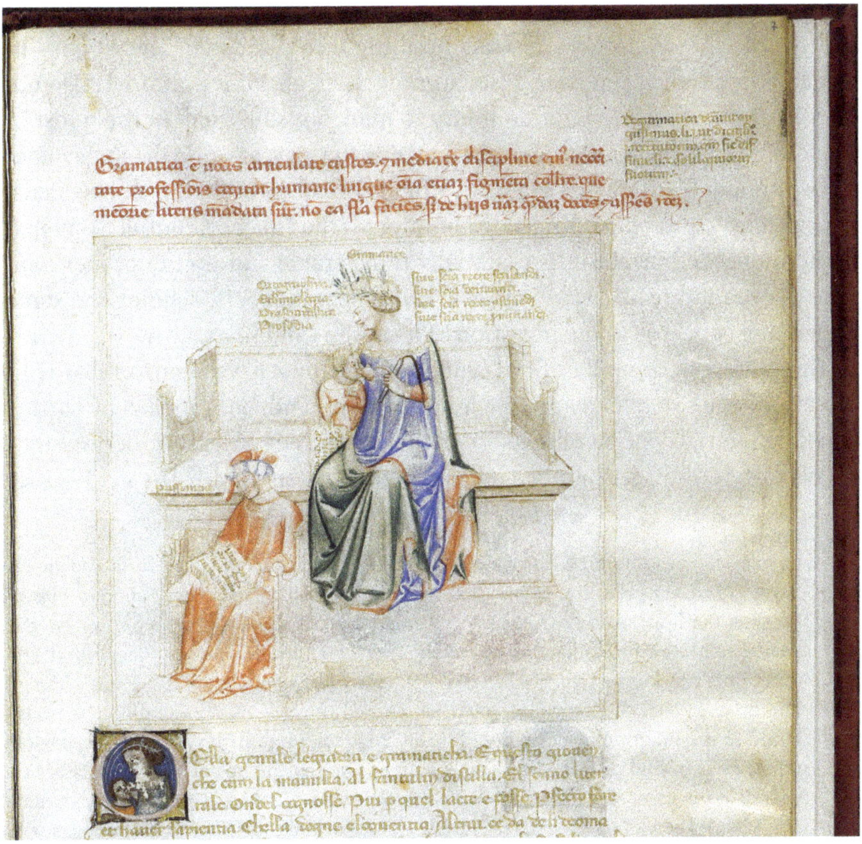

FIGURE 4 Grammar imparts her wisdom through nourishing milk, teaching her child the alphabet. Chantilly, Musée Condé, 0599 (1426), fol. 7r. Bibliothèque et archives du château de Chantilly

with a child learning the alphabet while nursed at her breast, underscoring the intertwined notions of instruction, embodiment, and nourishment.

Although at first glance distant from Columba's tale, this image arguably captures its underlying logic. It is fair to wonder whether the scribe who compiled the *Leabhar Breac* was consciously aware of the principles of sympathy and antipathy – or at least understood them implicitly. In the same manuscript, he includes the *Pais Iacoip apstail* – the *Passion of Saint James* – which appears to coincide with an earlier Latin text, the *Passio Iacobi*, found in the apocryphal *Acts of the Apostles* attributed to pseudo-Abdias, traditionally considered the first Bishop of Babylon, possibly dating to the sixth or seventh century.[56] In this

56 Reginald D. Pringle, "Traditions Relating to St James the Great in the Accounts of Medieval Latin Pilgrims to the Holy Land," in *Translating the Relics of St James: From Jerusalem to*

account, the Apostle James converts his adversaries, the magician Hermogenes and his disciple Philetus, and convinces them to dispose of their books of magic. When Hermogenes suggests burning them all, James cautions: "Do not do so, lest the smoke thereof do injury to men, but sink them in the midst of the sea."[57] Hermogenes complies, recognising the logic at work: the malevolent force contained within the volumes would spread through the smoke, causing harm by "contact." This narrative reinforces the concept, central to sympathetic thought, that power is materially transferable and that improper handling – even indirectly, as in smoke – can transmit effects, echoing the same underlying concerns as the ingestion of letters in Columba's story.

Therefore, the compiler of the *Leabhar Breac* must have been familiar with these principles.[58] In early and high medieval Ireland, both the act of writing and the material content of texts were often objects of veneration, a reverence largely fostered by Christianity, a religion of the written word.[59] The significance

---

Compostela, ed. Antón M. Pazos (Routledge, 2017), 123–39, at 123–4; Marta Ameijeiras Barros, "Rediscovering the Jacobean Cult in Medieval England: The Wall Paintings of St James the Great in Stoke Orchard," *Ad Limina* 6, no. 6 (2015): 221–49, at 237.

57 *The Passions and the Homilies from Leabhar Breac: Text, Translation and Glossary*, ed. and trans. Robert Atkinson (Hodges Figgis, 1887), 348.

58 The broader idea that language could be learned through supernatural means is also found in the tradition associated with Saint Brendan. In an Irish version of his hagiography, he asks God to teach him Greek instantly so that he might read the Missal in a church at the monastery of the monk Gildas, in Britain. His wish is immediately granted. *Life of Brendan of Clonfert*, in *Lives of Irish Saints*, ed. and trans. Charles Plummer, 2 vols. (Oxford University Press, 1922), II, 44–92, at 81. Something similar happens to St. Patrick, as we read in the *Leabhar Breac* in the preface to a hymn ascribed to Saint Sechnall (Secundinus), known as *Audite Omnes Amantes*. The preface provides some biographical information about the saint, including the following: when Patrick was newly born, he was brought to the blind priest Gorianas to be baptised. However, the priest had no water to administer the sacrament, and traced a cross on the ground with the child's hand: a spring of water gushed forth from that spot at once. The water had miraculous powers: Gorianas washed his face with it and instantly regained his sight, and became able to recite the readings to perform the baptism despite he had never learned to read. *Preface to the Hymn of St. Sechnall*, in *The Irish Liber Hymnorum*, ed. John H. Bernard and Robert Atkinson (Harrison and Sons, 1898), 3–13, at 4. In Irish vernacular tradition, the beautiful Eithne learns to read just after converting to Christianity. Anton Gerard van Hamel, "The Celtic Grail," *Revue Celtique* 47 (1930): 340–82, at 371; Borsje, "Druids, Deer and 'Words of Power,'" 40.

59 Sarah Künzler, *Flesh and Word. Reading Bodies in Old Norse-Icelandic and Early Irish Literature* (de Gruyter, 2016), 301–2; Ann Dooley, *Playing the Hero: Reading the Irish Saga Táin Bó Cúailnge* (University of Toronto Press, 2006), 24; Hildegard L.C. Tristram, "Feis und fled: Wirklichkeit und Darstellung in mittelalterlichen irischen Gastmahlserzählungen," in ead., ed., *Medialität und mittelalterliche insulare Literatur* (Narr, 1992), 183–220, at 189–90.

of the material body and its capacity to receive and embody "spiritual inscriptions" is attested throughout both the Old and New Testaments.[60]

Yet, the story of Columba's edible alphabet does not fit neatly within this *motif*.[61] There is little doubt alphabet-shaped cakes – or other foods, such as apples[62] – had long been used for educational purposes since antiquity.[63] In this sense, the author of the *Life of Columba* could rely on a solid and longstanding tradition of graphophagy with several potential functions, ranging from pedagogy to the symbolic ingestion of knowledge and power.

The origin of the scribe's story of the alphabet in the *Leabhar Breac* remains uncertain, although we know it was not included in the earlier lives of the saint. Its absence from preceding *vitae* and collections of *virtutes* indicates that this episode was a later addition to the hagiographic tradition. Consequently, we can infer that the narrative served a specific rhetorical purpose. After all, as with most elements in a hagiographic text – including miracles – each detail was carefully selected to convey meaning or reinforce the saint's exemplary character. The question, then, is why this particular passage, depicting the ingestion of letters, was inserted among the saint's remarkable deeds?

The episode of the alphabet inscribed on bread can thus be understood as a miracle – or rather, a double miracle. First, Columba acquires the ability to read instantaneously; second, his consumption of the bread prophetically enacts his destined role as the "dove of the Church" across two lands. It seems fair to conclude that, even if the author was inspired by widespread practices of teaching children the alphabet through edible letters, the event is deliberately suffused with a miraculous aura. The narrative leaves no room for ambiguity: this is not ordinary, but "miraculous" learning, entirely fitting with the expectations of a saintly life.

---

60 E.g., Deut 6:6; Rev 3:11–12. There are several examples, in the Bible, concerning the power of words. It suffices to recall God's act of creation, which takes place by means of naming things, and John's verse "In principio erat Verbum," where the Word is God himself (Jn 1:1). A few lines down, John writes that "the Word was made flesh," thus equating it with Christ (Jn 1:14). Consequently, it should not come as a surprise that Christian mentality attributed special power to language. Indeed, these verses were employed in a number of medical remedies.

61 On this motif, see Ernst R. Curtius, *European Literature and the Latin Middle Ages*, ed. Willard R. Trask, 7th ed. (Princeton University Press, 1990), 312.

62 Patricia A. Rosenmeyer, *Ancient Epistolary Fictions: The Letter in Greek Literature* (Cambridge University Press, 2001), 98–130; Elena Zaffagno, "Il giuramento scritto sulla mela," *Materiali e contributi per la storia della narrativa greca* 1 (1976): 109–19.

63 Peter Kruschwitz, "Writing on Trees: Restoring a Lost Facet of the Graeco-Roman Epigraphic Habit," *Zeitschrift für Papyrologie und Epigraphik* 173 (2010): 45–62, at 46.

In the Irish *Life of Columba* preserved in the *Leabhar Breac* and the *Book of Lismore*, the saint's acquisition of literacy occurs through unconventional means. However, the narrative does not invoke explicitly Christian supernatural powers; the only reference to a supernatural source points to a member of the ancient Celtic learned class: the *vatis*. It is the *vatis* who suggests that the alphabet be written, though he does not specify that it should be on a cake – the origin of this particular detail remains uncertain, though it seems to be attributed to the priest Cruithnechán. Regardless of the source, the outcome is immediate and unmistakable.

From this, some observations emerge:

1. The notion of sympathetic absorption was fully compatible with the hagiographer's understanding of the "supernatural";
2. This concept could be seamlessly integrated into an Irish hagiographic narrative;
3. It could be employed, even rhetorically, to commemorate a pivotal event in the life of a saint central to Irish Christianity;
4. The hagiographer evidently assumed that the audience would grasp the principle without confusion, suggesting either that it harmonised naturally with a Christian supernatural framework or that contemporaries did not regard its non-Christian origins – embodied in the figure of the *vatis* – as problematic.

As observed above, this continuity of beliefs and practices was shaped in large part by the cultural and social context of Ireland's Christianisation.[64] It is important to emphasise, however, that literary evidence of such practices is attested in other typologies of sources as well.

A notable example is the *Book of Durrow*, a manuscript preserved at Trinity College, Dublin, dating from the second half of the seventh century. Practical signs of how it was used are still visible. Produced in an Irish monastic *scriptorium* in or near Durrow in Count Offaly, Ireland, this vellum manuscript was preserved at the Abbey of Durrow from at least the eleventh century until the seventeenth.[65] As the oldest surviving fully illuminated Insular Gospel Book, it bears witness not only to artistic achievement but also to devotional practice. In the sixteenth century, after passing into private hands, it was borrowed and

64 Roger Powell, "The Book of Kells, the Book of Durrow. Comments on the vellum, the make-up and other aspects," *Scriptorium* 10, no.1 (1956): 3–21; Richard Johnson-Sheehan, Paul Lynch, "Rhetoric of Myth, Magic, and Conversion: A Prolegomena to Ancient Irish Rhetoric," *Rhetoric Review* 26, no. 3 (2007): 233–52, at 248.

65 Bernard Meehan, *The Book of Durrow: a medieval masterpiece at Trinity College Dublin* (Town House and Country House, 1996); Rijcklof Hofman, "Durrow, Book of," in *The Encyclopaedia of Ireland*, ed. Brian Lalor (Gill & Macmillan, 2003), 330.

studied by James Ussher, Bishop of Meath. Later, however, it came into the hands of some farmer who worshipped it as a relic of St. Columba and believed it possessed properties. To release these powers, he immersed the manuscript in water to make a potion intended to cure sick cattle. In the seventeenth century, Conell Mageoghagan recorded the "strange property" attributed to Columba's books,

> which is that if they or any of them had sunck to the bottom of the Deepest waters they would not lose one letter, signe, or character of them, wch I have seen partly myselfe of that book of them which is at Dorow in the K^{s} County, for I saw the Ignorant man that had the same in his Custody, when sickness came upon cattle, for their Remedy putt water on the booke & suffered it to rest there a while & saw alsoe cattle returne thereby to their former or pristin state & the book to receave no loss.[66]

The folios still bear the signs of the effect of the water on the ink (fig. 5): some leaves cockled, and some ink smudged.[67]

This episode recalls Bede's account of parchment scrapings used to prepare antidotes against snakes' venom. In such cases, the material object itself appears to have been more important than the specific textual content it bore. Although the manuscript contains the four Gospels alongside a number of prefatory texts – certainly susceptible to being regarded as inherently thaumaturgic – its alleged efficacy was instead attributed to the belief that St. Columba himself had been its original scribe.[68] Since late antiquity, the function of Gospels and their excerpts extended far beyond liturgical reading, as they served as talismans, oath-objects, and therapeutic substances.[69]

Such practices persisted in Ireland not because pagan elements survived Christianisation, but because Irish Christian culture maintained robust assumptions about materiality that made textual consumption theologically

66 Denis Murphy, ed., *The Annals of Clonmacknoise, being Annals of Ireland from the Earliest Period to A.D. 1408, translated into English A.D. 1627 by Conell Mageohegan* (Dublin University Press, 1896), 95–6.

67 This may be the same reason why some of the leaves of an earlier French manuscript, namely Dijon, Bibliothèque Municipale, MS 448 (dating from the eleventh or twelfth century) are also cockled and stained. Skemer, *Binding Words*, 256–7.

68 This idea was quite spread in early medieval Europe, Ireland included. Niamh Wycherley, *The Cult of Relics in Early Medieval Ireland*, Studies in the Early Middle Ages 43 (Brepols, 2015), 38.

69 Robert M. Calhoun, "The Gospel(-amulet) as God's Power for Salvation," *Early Christianity* 10 (2019): 21–55.

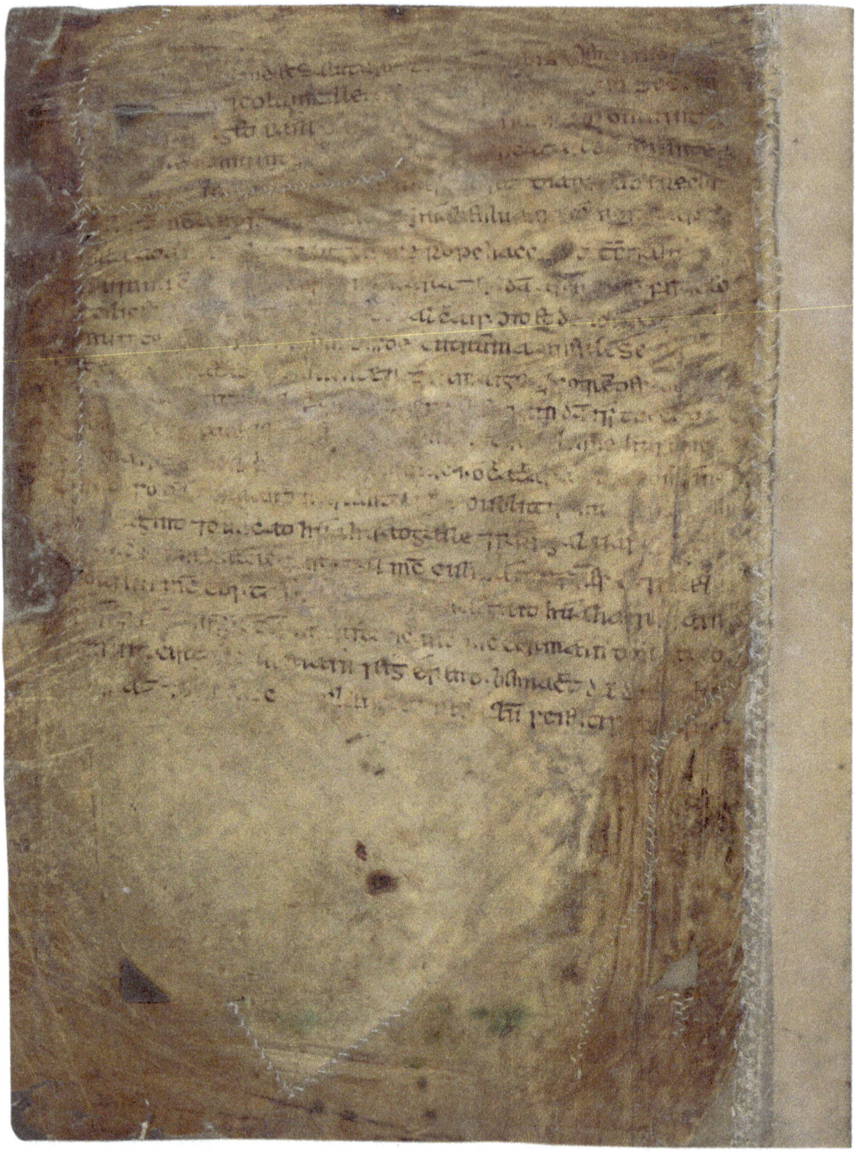

FIGURE 5 A smudged and crumpled page from the Book of Durrow clearly bearing the marks of water immersion, Dublin, Trinity College MS 57, fol. 248v (Source: the Board of Trinity College)

plausible and practically authoritative. This "materialism" preceded Christianity but was not essentially opposed to it; rather, Christian incarnational theology, Eucharistic realism, and relic veneration provided new justifications for what remained a consistent cultural orientation toward materialised power.[70] The *Book of Durrow* case illustrates this convergence: the manuscript's efficacy derived simultaneously from its association with St. Columba (relic logic), its textual content (Gospel power), and the material properties of vellum and ink (sympathetic logic). These categories were not competing explanations but mutually reinforcing aspects of a therapeutic system perceived as unified. Whatever the case, it appears that hagiographic tradition reflected actual beliefs that endured for centuries. This is corroborated by the abundant evidence preserved in leechbooks.[71]

An enduring continuity likely existed between Irish manuscripts and medical remedies and the vast *corpus* of early English medical collections, which themselves preserved a significant amount of older ritual and oral elements.[72] Deborah Hayden has described this process as the active transmission of medical learning across the Irish Sea, characterising it as "the participation of Irish writers in wider scholarly trends concerning the power of languages, cryptography, and obscurantist vocabulary prevalent in Canterbury and elsewhere in Europe prior to the twelfth century."[73]

---

70 Peter Brown, *The Cult of the Saints: Its Rise and Function in Latin Christianity* (The University of Chicago Press, 1981), 2; Carolyne Walker Bynum, "The Sacrality of Things: An Inquiry into Divine Materiality in the Christian Middle Ages," *Irish Theological Quarterly* 78, no. 1 (2012): 3–18.

71 On extant medieval Irish medical manuscripts, see Aoibheann Nic Dhonnchadha, "Medical Writing in Irish," *Irish Journal of Medical Science* 169 (2000): 217–20. See Deborah Hayden, "The Context and Obscure Language of Medical Charms in a Sixteenth-century Irish Remedy Book: Four Case Studies," in *Obscuritas in Medieval Irish and Welsh Literature*, ed. Chantal Kobel (forthcoming). See, for instance, Dublin, RIA MS 24 B 3, 92–93.

72 Deborah Hayden, "Old English in the Irish Charms," *Speculum* 97, no. 2 (2022): 349–76; Meaney, "Extra-medical Elements." The Irish medical corpus was also influenced by late-medieval Latin texts benefiting from Arabic medical tradition: Francis Shaw, "Medieval Medico-philosophical Treatises in the Irish Language," in *Féil-sgríbhinn Eóin Mhic Néill: Essays and Studies Presented to Professor Eoin MacNeill, D. Litt., on the Occasion of His Seventieth Birthday, May 15th 1938*, ed. John Ryan (Three Candles, 1940), 144–57.

73 Hayden, "Old English in the Irish Charms," 375. On the circulation of medical knowledge in Anglo-Saxon England, see also: Linda E. Voigts, "Anglo-Saxon Plant Remedies and the Anglo-Saxons," *Isis* 70 (1979): 250–68; Malcolm L. Cameron, *Anglo-Saxon Medicine* (Cambridge University Press, 1993), 100–58; Id., "Anglo-Saxon Medicine and Magic," *Anglo-Saxon England* 17 (1988): 191–215; Id., "Bald's *Leechbook* and Cultural Interactions in Anglo-Saxon England," *Anglo-Saxon England* 19 (1990): 5–12; Audrey L. Meaney, "The Practice of Medicine about the Year 1000," *Social History of Medicine* 13, no. 2 (2000): 221–37; Debby Banham, "Dun, Oxa and Pliny the Great Physician: Attribution

Examples from England are particularly striking. The texts that constitute the Old English *materia medica* – *Bald's Leechbook*,[74] *Leechbook III*,[75] the *Lacnunga*,[76] the *Old English Herbarium* and the *Medicina de Quadrupedibus* (the latter two commonly grouped together as the *Old English Pharmacopeia*[77]) – form the earliest collections of medical material in a Western vernacular and are therefore key resources for this study.[78] Even though each text has its own distinctive features, all draw to varying degrees on shared Latin and vernacular sources and belong to a broadly coherent tradition. They also display important affinities in terms of structure, aims, and underlying pharmaceutical principles. Chronologically speaking, *Bald's Leechbook* and *Leechbook III* are the earliest of these compilations, while the *Lacnunga* and the *Old English Pharmacopeia* date to the final phase of the Anglo-Saxon period.

A striking feature of the Old English medical collections is not the sheer presence of written words as therapeutic devices, but rather the highly circumscribed contents in which they are employed. Writing is mostly absent from remedies addressing ordinary physiological conditions, while it appears almost exclusively in treatment for fevers, demonic affliction, and illnesses attributed

---

and Authority in Old English Medical Texts," *Social History of Medicine* 24, no. 1 (2011): 57–73; Ead, "England Joins the Medical Mainstream: New Texts in Eleventh-Century Manuscripts," in *Anglo-Saxon England and the Continent*, ed. Hans Sauer and Joanna Story (Arizona Center for Medieval and Renaissance Studies, 2011), 341–51; Ead, "*Lectun* and *Orceard*: A Preliminary Survey of the Evidence for Horticulture in Anglo-Saxon England," in *The Anglo-Saxons: the World Through Their Eyes*, ed. Gale R.Owen-Crocker and Brian W. Schneider (Archaeopress, 2014), 33–48.

74 London, British Library Royal MS 12 D. xvii.

75 This collection, which bears the name given to it by Cockayne, is included in the same manuscript as *Bald's Leechbook*.

76 London, British Library Harley MS 585. Modern edition: Edward Pettit, *Anglo-Saxon Remedies, Charms, and Prayers from British Library MS Harley 585: The «Lacnunga»*, 2 vols. (The Edwin Mellen Press, 2001).

77 These two collections are the only ones to have been preserved in multiple manuscripts. Modern edition: *The Old English Herbarium and Medicina de Quadrupedibus*, ed. Hubert Jan De Vriend (Oxford University Press, 1984).

78 Emily Kesling, *Medical Texts in Anglo-Saxon Literary Culture* (D.S. Brewer, 2020), 1–22; Stephanie Hollis, "Scientific and Medical Writings," in *A Companion to Anglo-Saxon Literature*, ed. Phillip Pulsiano and Elaine Treharne (Blackwell, 2001), 188–208, at 194–205. The Old English medical collections were first edited by Oswald Cockayne: *Leechdoms, Wortcunning, and Starcraft of Early England, Being a Collection of Documents Illustrating the History of Science in this Country Before the Norman Conquest*, ed. and trans. Oswald Cockayne, 3 vols. (Longman, Green, Longman, Roberts, and Green, 1864–66; repr. Cambridge University Press, 2012), ii, books 1 and 2.

to elves or other non-human agents.[79] This pattern is not random but likely systematic. Writing was activated precisely when disease was conceptualised as exceeding the boundaries of the purely somatic, requiring forms of intervention capable of addressing invisible or morally charged causes.

For instance, in *Leechbook III*, the only remedy involving a written text is prescribed for *ælfsogoða* (an unspecified disease ascribed to elvish influence) and for the Devil's temptations.[80] The therapeutic sequence is carefully structured: a text with numerous Christian references is written down, then a series of prayers are sung over it and over a drink made from various herbs. The sign of the cross is drawn three times in the drink with oil of the sick (olive oil or another plant oil blessed by a bishop or a priest). Another sign of the cross is made with the writing over the drink, accompanied by a prayer to expel the devil from the patient's body. Eventually, the text is dipped in the drink and the sign of the cross is made with it on the patient's limbs. Whether or not the liquid was ultimately ingested is left unspecified, but this ambiguity is revealing in itself.[81] The remedy does not depend on ingestion as such; rather, it constructs a chain of ritual actions in which writing, prayer, gesture, and object interact to reorient the patient's condition. Writing here functions less as a pharmaceutical ingredient than as a catalyst within a broader performative framework.
A similar logic underlies an exorcism to cure fever in *Bald's Leechbook*, compiled around the late ninth century,[82] where John 1:1–3[83] is written on a sacramental paten along with symbolic signs: eighteen crosses and the letters A and Ω (fig. 6).[84]

The Alpha and Omega were references to God, derived from Revelation 1:8 ("I am Alpha and Omega"). The number of crosses may symbolically refer

79 Katherine Storm Hindley, "Text Over Time: The Written Word in English Charms Before 1350," *Incantatio* 7 (2018): 72–93, at 75.

80 London, British Library Royal MS 12 D. xvii, fols. 124v–125r.

81 Godfrid Storms, *Anglo-Saxon Magic* (Springer, 1948; Repr. 2013), 230.

82 The only complete edition and translation of the *Leechbook* remains Cockayne's. A more recent and rigorous critical edition is: Marilyn Deegan, *A Critical Edition of MS.B.L.Royal 12.D.xvii: Bald's Leechbook*, unpub. Ph.D. Diss. (University of Manchester, 1988). On this leechbook's intellectual context, see Malcolm L. Cameron, "The Sources of Medical Knowledge in Anglo-Saxon England," *Anglo-Saxon England* 11 (1982): 135–55; Id., "Bald's *Leechbook*: Its Sources and their Uses in its Compilation," *Anglo-Saxon England* 12 (1983): 153–82; Audrey L. Meaney, "Variant Versions of Old English Medical Remedies and the Compilation of Bald's Leechbook," *Anglo-Saxon England* 13 (1984): 235–68.

83 "In principio erat Verbum et Verbum erat apud Deum et Deus erat Verbum. Hoc erat in principio apud Deum omnia per ipsum facta sunt."

84 London, British Library Royal MS 12 D. xvii, fols. 51r–v. The letter omega is written in lowercase (ω), but in a way that makes it resemble "LD."

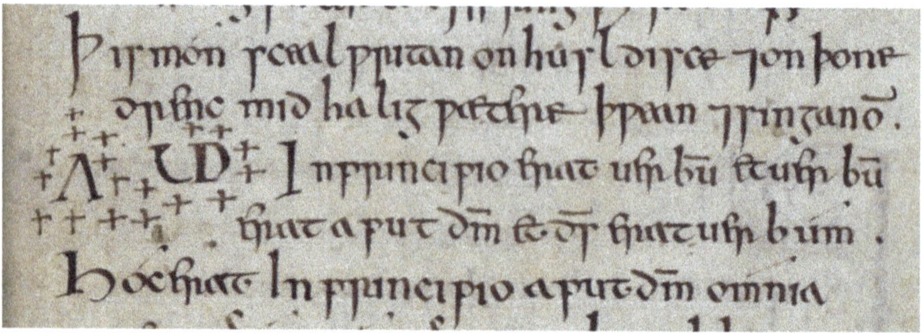

FIGURE 6 Symbolic references to God and to the Gospels were powerful ingredients in Anglo-Saxon medicine. London, British Library Royal MS 12 D. xvii, fol. 51r (Courtesy of the British Library)

to the concept of liberation: for example, the Israelites were oppressed by the Philistines and the Ammonites for eighteen years before being freed.[85] Alternatively, it might simply allude to Christ's miraculous healing of a woman who had been crippled by a spirit for eighteen years.[86] Finally, the verses come from Johannine prologue – scripture's most elevated statement about divine Word as cosmic principle.

The verses and diagram were then washed off the paten with holy water, which was collected in a cup. The ritual continued with the recitation of the Creed, the Lord's Prayer, Psalms 118 and 119 from the Vulgate, several lines from Sedulius's *Carmen Paschale*, and a Christian formula of exorcism against fever, invoking the Lord to drive the affliction out of the patient's body. Finally, both the patient and the physician were required to drink the holy water three times, now imbued with the power of the written and spoken formulas.

The precise symbolism of these elements is open to interpretation, but their cumulative effect is unequivocal: the configuration locates the illness within a narrative of divine authority and liberation. The written text is not preserved as a stable artefact, and thus the efficacy of the remedy does not reside in any single component, but in the progressive transformation of words into action and substance. The remedy presumes that the Word's creative power, celebrated in John's Gospel, can be activated through inscription, dissolution, and ingestion. Analogical thought treated cosmic and somatic as structurally parallel, each reflecting divine order at different scales.

85 Jdg 10:8.

86 Lk 13:11–13. It is worth noting that, in Jewish tradition, eighteen is the numerical value of *chai* ("life"), making it an auspicious number – though this would hardly have influenced the compiler.

The *Lacnunga*, preserved in a manuscript compiled between the end of the tenth and the early eleventh century,[87] develops this approach further by embedding writing within highly elaborate ritual procedures. A remedy against *ælfsiden* and *feondes costunga*,[88] that is, intended to counteract all harm caused by elves and the devil, requires Gospel passages ("In principio erat verbum …"), psalms, and prayers to be written, dissolved into liquid, combined with herbs and consecrated wine, and subjected to multiple masses.[89] Here writing is one step in a process of ritual intensification, repeatedly reframed through liturgical performance. Moreover, its power is enhanced by means of ritual tools that may have been believed themselves to possess powers, such as wine and the paten.[90] At the same time, the manuscript makes clear that writing was not indispensable for activating linguistic power. Several remedies rely exclusively on spoken formulas, which are sung not only over ingredients but also directly into the patient's mouth, ears, or wounds.[91] In such cases, the voice itself becomes the medium through which language is made operative, suggesting that the distinction between written and spoken words was functionally secondary to their correct ritual deployment.

One such remedy is the well-known "Nine Herbs Charm."[92] This charm blends practical herbal medicine with pagan and Christian influences, invoking nine specific plants – mugwort, plantain open to the east, lamb's cress, betony, mayweed, nettle, wild sour apple, thyme or chervil, and fennel – alongside prayers and ritual actions to treat poison and infections.[93] The plants were grounded into powder, mixed with the soap and the pulp of the apple. Then, a paste of water and ashes was to be prepared and boiled with fennel. The charm (*galdor*) was to be sung over the plants and the apple three times before they

87 On the text's intellectual context, see: Karen L. Jolly, *Popular Religion in Late Saxon England: Elf Charms in Context* (University of North Carolina Press, 1996), 107; Meaney, "Extra-medical Elements," esp. 51ff; Cameron, *Anglo-Saxon Medicine*, 34ff.

88 On these terms, see Alaric Hall, *Elves in Anglo-Saxon England: Matters of Belief, Health, Gender and Identity* (Boydell Press, 2007).

89 Pettit, *Anglo-Saxon Remedies*, i, 17, no. 29.

90 See, for instance, Megan Cavell, "Powerful Patens in the Anglo-Saxon Medical Tradition and Exeter Book Riddle 48," *Neophilologus* 101, no. 1 (2017): 129–38.

91 Pettit, *Anglo-Saxon Remedies*, i, 37, no. 64. On the issues concerning the ending of entry no. 63 and the beginning of entry no. 64, see Pettit, *Anglo-Saxon Remedies*, ii, 61–2. For other examples, see ibid., i, 115, no. 164 and 165.

92 Ibid., ii, 98ff.

93 On the herbs and the context of the charm, Debby Banham, "The Old English Nine Herbs Charm," in *Medieval Christianity in Practice*, ed. Miri Rubin (Princeton University Press, 2009), 189–93.

were prepared, and also "into the mouth and both ears and into the wounds" of the patient, before applying the salve on it.[94]

Later evidence confirms the persistence and adaptability of this logic. Remedies prescribing inscribed sacramental wafers or other foodstuffs appear from the eleventh century onward, particularly in treatments for fever and childbirth. For example, on the *verso* of the fly-leaf at the end of a manuscript preserved at the Worcester Cathedral Library, likely copied between ca. 1030 and 1070, one finds a cure for fever reading: "genim .ix. oflætan ⁊ gewrit on ælcere on þas wisan: ies*us* chr*istus*" ("Take nine sacramental wafers and write on each one in this way: ies*us* chr*istus*").[95] Moreover, nine Lord's prayers were to be chanted over them, after which the patient would consume three wafers daily for three consecutive days. Each day, an adjuration formula was recited over the patient, invoking the Holy Trinity, the Seven Sleepers of Ephesus, and other Christian figures such as the Evangelists. Through this formula, the fever and chills were commanded to depart from the afflicted person's body: "coniuro vos, frigora et febres [...] adiuro [...] vos diabolicum [...] non habe [...] ullum [...] malum."[96] As evidenced by the structured phases of the healing process and the requirement for wafers, the involvement of a churchman was indispensable.

Hosts could be either consecrated or not, depending on the case. It could be supposed that they usually were, since they were attributed special powers possibly as they were thought to embody divinity. However, this posed a series of practical problems, such as the availability of consecrated wafers for use outside of Mass.[97] The use of hosts was not forbidden according to theological texts from late Anglo-Saxon England, which suggests that clerical participation was implied. The Church placed particular emphasis on ensuring proper handling of the Corpus Christi. Already in the early medieval period, guidelines were established for dealing with unconsumed hosts: they were to be either consumed by the ministers or burned, with the ashes carefully disposed of. This issue gained greater significance from the eleventh century

94 Ibid., i, 76, no. 69.

95 Worcester Cathedral Library, Ms Q.5. The manuscript was transcribed in Arthur S. Napier, "Altenglische Miscellen," *Archiv für das Studium der neueren Sprachen und Literaturen* 83, no. 4 (1890): 323–27, at 324. The manuscript includes works by Bede and Priscian and is mostly focused on grammar.

96 On dwarves and elves in Anglo-Saxon medicine, see Lotte Motz, "Of Elves and Dwarfs," *Arv: Journal of Scandinavian Folklore* 29–30 (1973–74): 93–127; Conan Doyle, "*Dweorg* in Old English: Aspects of Disease Terminology," *Quaestio Insularis* 9 (2008): 99–117.

97 Lea T. Olsan, "Writing on the Hand in Ink: A Late Medieval Innovation in Fever Charms in England," *Incantatio* 7 (2018): 9–45, at 31.

onward, as concerns grew about the misuse of sacramental wafers for superstitious purposes, a problem that became especially pronounced after the twelfth century.[98]

Monks and churchmen providing medical care transmitted remedies involving inscribed bread for different purposes.[99] They could help with childbirth, for instance: a remedy contained in Sloane MS 475, dating from the first quarter of the twelfth century, suggests inscribing specific *caracteres* on the crust of common bread, and feeding it to the pregnant woman (fig. 7).[100] The remedy is included in the first part of the manuscript, which was produced in England in the early twelfth century and was likely the personal book of a medical practitioner. It contains medical recipes, charms, a few medical treatises and prognostics. The aforementioned prescription is immediately followed by another graphophagic one having the same purpose, reading: "On a cup write the letters *sator arepo tenet opera rotas*, and once they have been dissolved, she shall drink them with wine."[101] Unfortunately, no explanation is given concerning the composition of the ink. It is also possible that the words were carved into

98 *Paenitentiale Merseburgense a* (*recensio W10*), in *Paenitentialia minora Franciae et Italiae*, ed. Raymund Kottje, CCSL 156 (Brepols, 1994), 126–64, c. 48; Regino of Prüm, *Libri duo de synodalibus causis et disciplinis ecclesiasticis*, ed. Friedrich G.A. Wasserschleben (Akademische Druck- u. Verlagsanstalt, 1964 [1840]) i, 71, 56; *Poenitentiale Valicellanum III*, in *Die Bussordnungen der abendländischen Kirche nebst einer rechtsgeschichtlichen Einleitung*, ed. Friedrich Wilhelm Hermann Wasserschleben (Ch. Graeger, 1851; repr. 1958), 682–88, c. 10, 686. See Peter Browe, "Die Eucharistie als Zaubermittel im Mittelalter," *Archiv für Kulturgeschichte* 20 (1930): 134–54; Id., *Die eucharistischen Wunder des Mittelalters* (Müller und Seiffert, 1938); Jesús Montoya Martínez, "El culto a la Eucaristía y sus derivaciones mágicas en el siglo XIII," *La corónica: A Journal of Medieval Hispanic Languages, Literatures, and Cultures* 36, no. 1 (2007): 189–96; Andrea Maraschi, "Sympathy for the Lord: The Host and Elements of Sympathetic Magic in Late Medieval Exempla," *Journal of Medieval Religious Cultures* 43, no. 2 (2017): 209–30.

99 Tony Hunt, *Popular Medicine in Thirteenth-Century England. Introduction and Texts* (Boydell&Brewer, 1990); Peter Murray Jones and Lea T. Olsan, "Performative Rituals for Conception and Childbirth in England, 900–1500," *Bulletin of the History of Medicine* 89, no. 3 (2015): 406–33. Among other things, in the tenth century, a *Benedictio salis et aque uel panis uel pomi uel casei* was used for fevers and chills. Adolph Franz, *Die kirchlichen Benediktionen im Mittelalter*, 2 vols. (Herdersche Verlagshandlung, 1909; repr. Akademische Druck und Verlagsanstalt, 1960), ii, 477–8.

100 London, British Library, Sloane MS 475, fol. 23r: "It*em* Fac hos caract*er*es in cr*us*tula panis. ⁊ fac mulieri comede*re*." On this and other similar cases, see Andrea Maraschi, "Writing on Bread. Remarks on Cultural and Practical Boundaries Starting from a Fourteenth-Century Commonplace Book," in *Medieval Borders and the Environment*, ed. Elisa Ramazzina (Brill, forthcoming).

101 London, British Library, Sloane MS 475, fol. 23r: "It*em* in scipho scribeas litt*er*as Sator arepo tenet op*er*a rotas et deletas bib*et* *cum* uino."

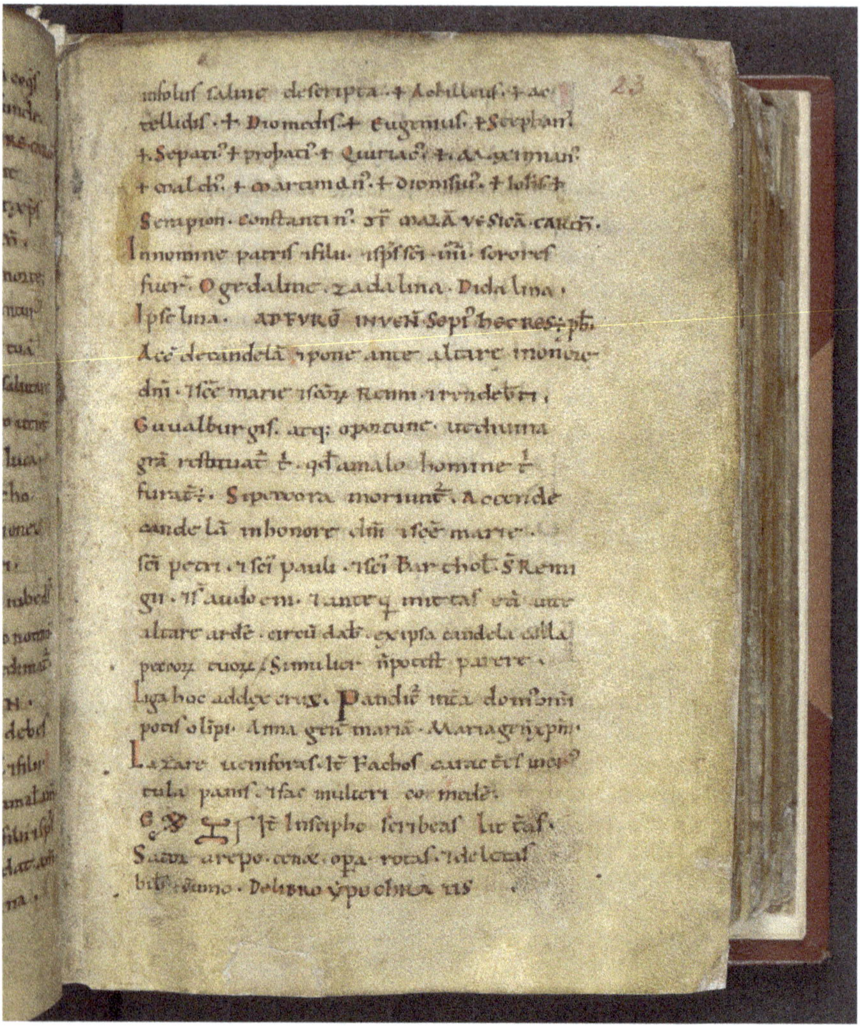

FIGURE 7 The last two remedies in this folio are two examples of graphophagy: words to eat on bread, and words to drink in wine. London, British Library, Sloane MS 475, fol. 23r. From the British Library's Collection

the interior of the cup, as material evidence from inscribed bowls discussed in this book suggests.

Remedies of this kind circulated for centuries, their efficacy and authority being reiterated in several manuscripts. For instance, the same recipe can be found in a fourteenth-century English manuscript: "Si mulier laboret in partu, sribe in pane uel in caseo Ogor Secor Vagor. Exi foras. In nomine patris etc."[102] In a later medical manuscript, butter replaces bread and the words to write on the food are again "sator arrepo [*sic*] tenet opera rotas".[103] In manuscript Sloane 475 there also appears a *carmen* for fever, which requires the practitioner to recite the Pater Noster and the patient to drink the names of the Seven Sleepers of Ephesus written in sage leaves in a sort of graphophagic decoction.[104] From the same period, in the benedictine abbey of Murbach in southern Alsace, a similar remedy appears in the medical scroll known as Rotulus von Mülinen.[105]

The types of food chosen were often selected based on the texture of their surface – either sufficiently hard or adequately soft – to allow for the inscription of letters: mostly butter, cheese, leek, apple, bread, sage leaves.[106] The efficacy of sacramental wafers was further enhanced by their symbolic significance. Sage may have been attributed special powers in part through its name – *salvia*, similar to *salvus*, "safe" and "saved." In the famous medical poem known as *Regimen sanitatis salernitatum*, believed to have been composed at the Schola Medica Salernitana between the twelfth and the thirteenth century – although some sources suggest it might date from the half of the eleventh century – sage is defined as "salvatrix" and "naturae conciliatrix."[107] The practice of inscribing

102 London, British Library, Sloane MS 3564, fol. 55r–v.

103 London, British Library, Egerton MS 833, f. 10r.

104 London, British Library, Sloane MS 475, fols. 22v–23r. The names are: "+ Achilleus. + actellidis. + Diomedis. + Eugenius. + Stephan*us*. + Sepati*us*. + probati*us*. + Quiriac*us*. + maximian*us*. + malch*us*. + martinian*us*. + dionisius. + Ioh*annis*. + Serapio. Constantin*us*." On the occurrence of these names in early English manuscripts, see Olsan, "Writing on the Hand in Ink." The *Lacnunga* recommends writing the seven names on seven sacramental wafers to cure fever. Here, however, the wafers are to be hung around the patient's neck (Pettit, *Anglo-Saxon Remedies*, i, 73, no. 86). See Jonathan Roper, *Charms and Charming in Europe* (Springer, 2004) 32–46. On this manuscript, see Norbert Kössinger, *Schriftrollen. Untersuchungen zu deutschsprachigen und mittelniederländischen Rotuli* (Reichert Verlag, 2020), 86–182; Walter Henzen, "Der Rotulus von Mülinen. Codex 803 der Burgerbibliothek Bern," in *Geschichte, Deutung, Kritik: Literaturwissenschaftliche Beiträge dargebracht zum 65. Geburtstag Werner Kohlschmidts*, ed. Maria Bindschedler and Paul Zinsli (Francke, 1969), 13–27.

105 Bern, Burgerbibliothek, Cod. 803, fol. 1r: "Ad febre*m*. Scribe hec nomina in una oblatione et da ad manducandu*m* ..."

106 For instance, in the eleventh-century manuscript Vatican City, Biblioteca Apostolica Vaticana, Barb. lat. 160, fol. 142r, a remedy for fever recommends writing certain "litteras in folias porri," which the patient should then eat.

107 *Das Medizinische Lehrgedicht der Hohen Schule zu Salerno: Regimen sanitatis Salerni*, ed. Paul Tesdorpf and Therese Tesdorpf-Sickenberger (Verlag von W. Kolhammer, 1915), lviii.

words on sage leaves – as well as on apples and wafers – to treat fever would be condemned by Bernardino of Siena in his *De idolatriae cultu*.[108]

Certain foods were favourite over others depending on the disease, but this comparative perspective can only be made when considering a wider chronological range. All in all, graphophagic remedies seems to have been relatively marginal in England until the second half of the eleventh century. Furthermore, food with inscribed formulae was not always meant to be eaten but also carried as amulet.[109]

The efficacy of oral formulas alone, even when written words were not a part of the recipes, represented another fundamental resource.[110] It would be overwhelming to look into all cases when spoken words were used to enrich the power of ingredients, or at least to make them fit for use in the right contexts. For instance, *Bald's Leechbook* instructs to sing masses over some herbs used to make a drink against lent addle or typhus fever. The herbs were then drenched with ale and the cocktail was boiled with the addition of holy water. When ready, as the patient drank the potion, the practitioner should say the names of the four evangelists, a charm, a prayer and more.[111] Or, against venom, the same leechbook suggests taking a Friday churn butter which had been milked from a female deer or cow of one colour, over which one should sing nine times a litany, the Pater Noster, and a charm.[112] It is not specified whether the butter was intended for consumption by the patient, but it is fair to assume so. In such cases, words were deemed a fundamental addition to the recipes, and were thought to be integral to the act of ingestion.[113]

108 "Contra febrem continuam, tertianam vel quartanam, dant herbarum folia scripta ad comedendum ieiunio stomacho, vel pomum scriptum sive scriptam hostiam, et hoc tribus diebus …". See Marina Montesano, *«Supra acqua et supra vento». "Superstizioni,"* maleficia *e* incantamenta *nei predicatori francescani osservanti (Italia, sec. XV)* (Istituto Storico Italiano per il Medio Evo, 1999), 64.

109 Hindley, "Eating Words and Burning Them," 362.

110 On the circulation of oral charms, see: Lea T. Olsan, "Charms and Prayers in Medieval Medical Theory and Practice," *Social History of Medicine* 16, no. 3 (2003): 343–66; Michael McVaugh, "Incantationes in Late Medieval Surgery," in *Ratio et Superstitio: Essays in Honor of Graziella Federici Vescovini*, ed. Giancarlo Marchetti, Orsolo Rignani, and Valeria Sorge (Fédération Internationale des Instituts d'Études Médiévales, 2003), 319–45.

111 London, British Library Royal MS 12 D. xvii, fol. 53r.

112 Ibid., fol. 43r. On colours in such context, see Wilfrid Bonser, "The Significance of Colour in Ancient and Mediaeval Magic: With Some Modern Comparisons," *Man* 25 (1925): 194–98.

113 Prayers and masses were crucial in a number of circumstances: when preparing a drink against demonic possession – e.g., London, British Library Royal MS 12 D. xvii, fols. 51v–52r; the mid-tenth-century *Pontificale Romano-Germanicum* took the utmost care to the regimen of the possessed: *Le Pontifical romano-germanique du dixième siècle*, ed. Cyrille Vogel

These descriptions also raise the question of which practitioner could have used similar texts. Scholars have suggested that practitioners were likely trained subjects who were part of educated circles, even though vernacular language used in texts might indicate a larger circulation.[114] It has been proposed that practitioners were both lay and ecclesiastical physicians, literate and illiterate, even though monastic centres and monks were likely protagonists in the practice of medicine and transmission of medical knowledge.[115] Emily Kesling has noted that the most important early English medical collections "continuously demonstrate their connections to intellectual culture and monasticism rather than lay practice."[116] They correlate with medical texts copied in Carolingian monasteries and "may have come to England through Carolingian channels."[117]

---

and Reinhard Elze, 3 vols. (Biblioteca Apostolica Vaticana, 1963), ii, 220–1 – or against *leod*-runes, to ease the digestion of meat – London, British Library Royal MS 12 D. xvii, fol. 53v – or to cure jaundice – ibid., fol. 107v. Potions against all temptations of the devil and to treat ailments related to *ælfe* ("elves") are similarly prepared with the aid of nine sung masses in *Leechbook III* (Ibid., fols. 120r–v; fols. 123v–124r; fols. 125v–126r). See Karen L. Jolly, "Anglo-Saxon Charms in the Context of a Christian World View," *Journal of Medieval History* 11 (1985): 279–93; Ead., "Magic, Miracle, and Popular Practice in the Early Medieval West: Anglo-Saxon England," in *Religion, Science and Magic in Concert and in Conflict*, ed. Jacob Neusner, Ernest S. Fredrichs, and Paul Virgil McCraken Flesher (Oxford University Press, 1989), 166–82; Ead., "Tapping the Power of the Cross: Who and for Who?," in *The Place of the Cross in Anglo-Saxon England*, ed. Catherine E. Karkov, Sarah L. Keefer, and Karen L. Jolly (The Boydell Press, 2006), 58–79. On *leodrunan*, see Kesling, *Medical Texts*, 61–2.

114 Meaney, "The Practice of Medicine"; Anne Van Arsdall, "Medical Training in Anglo-Saxon England," in *Form and Content of Instruction in Anglo-Saxon England in the Light of Contemporary Manuscript Evidence: Papers Presented at the International Conference*, Udine, 6–8 April 2006, ed. Patrizia Lendinara, Loredana Lazzari, and Maria Amalia D'Aronco (Brepols, 2007), 415–35; Debby Banham and Christine Voth, "The Diagnosis and Treatment of Wounds in the Old English Medical Collections: Anglo-Saxon Surgery?," in *Wounds and Wound Repair in Medieval Culture*, ed. Kelly DeVries and Larissa Tracey (Brill, 2015), 153–74.

115 Cameron, *Anglo-Saxon Medicine*, 19–24; Meaney, "The Practice of Medicine"; Anne Van Arsdall, "The Transmission of Knowledge in Early Medieval Medical Texts: An Exploration," in *Between Text and Patient: The Medical Enterprise in Medieval and Early Modern Europe*, ed. Florence Eliza Glaze and Brian K. Nance (SISMEL – Edizioni del Galluzzo, 2011), 201–15; Maria Amalia D'Aronco, "Anglo Saxon Plant Pharmacy and the Latin Medical Tradition," in *From Earth to Art: The Many Aspects of the Plant-World in Anglo-Saxon England. Proceedings of the First ASPNS Symposium,* University of Glasgow, 5–7 April 2000, ed. Carole P. Biggam (Rodopi, 2003), 133–51; Ead., "The Transmission of Medical Knowledge in Anglo- Saxon England: The Voices of Manuscripts," in *Form and Content of Instruction*, 35–58.

116 Kesling, *Medical Texts*, 3.

117 Ibid., 13. See also Maria Amalia D'Aronco, "L'erbario anglosassone, un'ipotesi sulla data della traduzione," *Romanobarbarica* 13 (1994/95): 325–66.

At least in the case of written formulas, practitioners were supposed to be educated, in that writing was not a technical skill widely available. In contrast, spoken formulas could be used by all those who happened to listen to them and memorise them, whether or not they understood their meaning. All in all, continuities between wide ranges of the social spectrum should not be ruled out.[118]

The aforementioned recipes show remarkable stability across centuries, even as the materials and inscriptions vary. What remains constant is the assumption that certain conditions demand forms of healing in which language must be physically or ritually integrated into the therapeutic process. Their authority seems to have rested instead on repetition, tradition, and successful performance. Taken together, these texts define a medical culture in which writing was neither ubiquitous nor marginal, but strategically reserved for situations where ordinary remedies seemed insufficient. When illness was thought to depend on hostile agencies, spiritual imbalance, or invisible forces, language became the go-to means of intervention. The remedies do not articulate a theoretical distinction between natural and supernatural medicine; rather, they operate within a continuum in which words, gestures, substances, and liturgy all shaped therapeutic efficacy.

It thus seems that Ireland and Britain represented cultural areas where graphophagy progressively spread and gained authority, and was eventually included in hagiographies and leechbooks, among others. The sources suggest that, in these regions, the power of language was activated through practice rather than doctrine. The persistence of these remedies across manuscripts, regions, and centuries suggests that they were not perceived as anomalous, but rather that Christianity progressively integrated ancient and popular practices into learned medicine.

118 Hindley, *Textual Magic*, 1–8. Cf. Carl Watkins, "'Folklore' and 'Popular Religion' in Britain during the Middle Ages," *Folklore* 115, no. 2 (2004): 140–50.

CHAPTER 3

The Merovingian, Carolingian, and Post-Carolingian World: Lost for Words?

Unlike what has been observed across the English Channel, tracing evidence of graphophagy in continental Europe proves considerably more challenging. This difficulty stems not only from the uneven survival of primary sources, but also from the intrinsic complexity of the phenomenon under investigation. The comparative scarcity does not necessarily indicate that such practices were less common in Francia than in Britain; it may instead reflect different manuscript cultures, distinct approaches to recording medical knowledge, or varying attitudes toward preserving recipes that occupied ambiguous religious and social positions.

Although several texts of diverse typologies were produced in Merovingian Gaul,[1] medicine did not constitute a particularly attractive field. Evidence of the existence of trained physicians enjoying high social status is counterbalanced by the scant number of medical treatises and recipe collections. Merovingian medical books, however, were not passive copies of texts drawn from Hippocratic and Galenic traditions: new handbooks of practical medicines were produced, rearranging such ancient knowledge. Studies of extant manuscripts reveal that medical knowledge was neither absent nor marginal but part of a wider manuscript culture that combined technical interests with generalist learning. Medical texts were present in miscellanies alongside other genres and compilers adapted and reworked material from late antiquity into new forms suited to contemporary readers. This continuity and transformation challenges older narratives that portray the early medieval West as hostile to medicine and suggests that medical knowledge participated in intellectual discourses well before the Carolingian reforms.[2]

A diverse range of texts from the period hint at an enduring anxiety about hunger, precarious health, feuds, and more, explaining the frequent recourse

1 Ian Wood, "The problem of late Merovingian culture," in *Exzerpieren – Kompilieren – Tradieren: Transformationen des Wissens zwischen Spätantike und Frühmittelalter*, ed. Stephan Dusil, Gerald Schwedler, and Raphael Schwitter (de Gruyter, 2017), 199–222, esp. 199–200.

2 James T. Palmer, "Merovingian Medicine Between Practical Art and Philosophy," *Traditio* 89 (2023): 17–45; Id., *Merovingian Worlds* (Cambridge University Press, 2025), 173–207.

 | HTTPS://DOI.ORG/10.1163/9789004765528-005

to supernatural solutions.[3] According to Gregory of Tours, both peasants and *potentes* relied on potions, ligatures, incantations, soothsayers and lots against demonic possessions, diseases, and to know the future.[4] This is not because they dared relying on the remnants of pagan rituals and reject Christianity, but rather these practices were likely part of lived Merovingian religion. "Grounded in religion," William Klingshirn has observed, "[…] these ideas and techniques relied for success on the widespread belief, not diminished by Christianity, that divine assistance was readily available, either directly or mediated through nature."[5]

Characters, special words, and formulae of various kinds were obviously part of this repertoire of techniques, as suggested in some sixth-century sermons by the bishop of Arles, Caesarius.[6] A homily composed in the second half of

3 William E. Klingshirn, "Magic and Divination in the Merovingian World," in *The Oxford Handbook of the Merovingian World*, ed. Bonnie Effros and Isabel Moreira (Oxford University Press, 2020), 968–87, at 969–70.

4 Gregory of Tours, *De virtutibus sancti Martini episcopi*, ed. Bruno Krusch, MGH SSRM 1.2 (Hahn, 1885), 134–211, 1.26–27 and 4.36; Gregory of Tours, *De passione et virtutibus sancti Juliani martyris*, ed. Bruno Krusch, MGH SSRM 1.2 (Hahn, 1885), 112–134, 46a; Gregory of Tours, *Historiarum libri decem*, ed. Bruno Krusch and Wilhelm Levison, MGH SSRM 1.1 (Hahn, 1937–1951), 9.10. On Merovingian medicine, see also: Valerie I.J. Flint, "The Early Medieval *medicus*, the Saint – and the Enchanter," *Social History of Medicine* 2, no. 2 (1989): 127–45; Edward James, "A Sense of Wonder: Gregory of Tours, Medicine, and Science," in *The Culture of Christendom. Essays in Medieval History in Commemoration of Denis L.T. Bethell*, ed. Marc A. Meyer (Hambledon Press, 1993), 45–60.

5 Klingshirn, "Magic and Divination," 968.

6 *Sancti Caesarii Arelatensis Sermones*, ed. Germain Morin, CCSL 103–104 (Brepols, 1953), 52.5: "let us offer some magical characters, let us affix some spells to his neck …"; 184.4: "if you had wanted to affix those characters to yourself, you could be healed …". Before Caesarius, Augustine, who laid the foundations for the discussion and critique of medieval magic, had already addressed as "superstitious" all the "bindings and remedies that even the discipline of physicians condemns, whether in incantations, in certain symbols – called characters – or in various objects to be suspended, tied, or even, in some way, danced about. These are not aimed at balancing the body but are directed toward certain meanings, whether hidden or manifest" ("omnes etiam ligaturae atque remedia, quae medicorum quoque disciplina condemnat, siue in praecantationibus siue in quibusdam notis, quos caracteres uocant, siue in quibusque rebus suspendendis atque inligandis uel etiam saltandis quodammodo, non ad temperationem corporum, sed ad quasdam significationes aut occultas aut etiam manifestas"). Augustine of Hippo, *De doctrina christiana*, ed. Joseph Martin, CCSL 32 (Brepols, 1962), ii, 19 (translation mine). He mentions the use characters in one of his sermons as well: "When he has a headache, he ties characters around his neck; and the one who does not want to die ties them around his neck as well" ("et quando illi caput dolet, caracteres sibi ad collum ligat; et qui non uult mori, ad collum sibi ligat"). Augustine of Hippo, *Sermones ad populum*, in *Sancti Augustini Sermones post Maurinos reperti*, ed. Germain Morin, *Miscellanea Agostiniana*, vol. 1 (Tipografia Poliglotta Vaticana, 1930), sermo 260D, 500.

the eighth century by an anonymous Frankish cleric in Alamannia or Raetia, preserved in a manuscript featuring a large collection of sermons and pastoral texts, mentions *carmina aut incantationes paganorum*, which were recited to cope with several different ailments and issues. It cautions against the use of written amulets and the imbibing of "a small drink with an incantation."[7] This is an important example, among others mentioned in the homily, of the powers attributed to *caracteria* and *scripturas*, which also included writing inscribed on papyrus, parchment, copper, iron or lead tablets, often to be hung around a person's or an animal's neck.[8]

It is hard to determine how widespread the practice of imbuing potions with oral incantations was, but evidence does indicate that the other types of amulets mentioned were indeed in use.[9] The two earliest surviving copies of Marcellus Empiricus' *De medicamentis*, an influential fifth-century medical text mingling Graeco-Roman and Gaulish popular medicine, were produced at Carolingian monasteries in the ninth century.[10] Marcellus's text represents a crucial moment in the textual preservation of vernacular healing, as it records local remedies, including numerous charms, into respectable Latin medical literature.[11] The manuscript tradition's persistence into Carolingian *scriptoria* reveals that monastic copyists found Marcellus's remedies – including graphophagic ones – compatible with Christian medicine.

7 Einsiedeln, Stiftsbibliotheck MS 281, 101–8. Edited in: *Homilia de sacrilegiis*, ed. Carl P. Caspari, in *Eine Augustin fälschlich beilegte Homilia de sacrilegiis* (Jacob Dybwad, 1886), 9, iv.15: "aliquid paruum cum incantatione bibit …". On this text's historical reliability, Yitzhak Hen, "The Early Medieval West," in *The Cambridge History of Magic and Witchcraft in the West: From Antiquity to the Present*, ed. David J. Collins (Cambridge University Press, 2015), 183–206, at 185–6.

8 *Homilia de sacrilegiis*, 11, vi.19. On these writing materials see Franco Cardini, "Il 'breve' (secoli XIV–XV): tipologia e funzione," *La Ricerca Folklorica* 5 (1982): 63–73, esp. 65. Importations of papyrus from the other side of the Mediterranean sea gradually stopped by the onset of the Carolingian period.

9 Ildar Garipzanov, "Magical Charaktêres in the Carolingian World: A Ninth-Century Charm in MS Vat. lat. 5359 and Its Broader Cultural Context," *Speculum* 96, no. 2 (2021): 287–308, at 302–3.

10 Respectively, Paris, BNF, MS Latin 6880 and Laon, Bibliothèque municipal, MS 420. Edited in: Marcellus Empiricus, *De Medicamentis Liber*, ed. Maximilian Niedermann, trans. Jutta Kollesch and Diethard Nickel, 2nd ed. (Akademie-Verlag, 1968). On the circulation of Marcellus Empiricus' work, see *Texts and Transmissions: A Survey of Latin Classics*, ed. Leighton D. Reynolds (Clarendon Press, 1983), 352–3. On the context preceding and surrounding Merovingian medicine, see Palmer, "Merovingian Medicine," 21ff.

11 Vivian Nutton, "From Medical Certainty to Medical Amulets: Three Aspects of Ancient Therapeutics," *Essays in the History of Therapeutics*, ed. Carolyne Walker Bynum and Vivian Nutton (Brill, 1991), 13–22.

The manuscripts include remedies employing the powers of Latin incantations, gibberish, formulas with Greek characters, often to be inscribed on lamellas of various materials and on fragments of papyrus, and to be hung around the neck or tied to the body.[12] Despite the Church's effort to oppose the use of amulets and beliefs in the efficacy of non-Christian formulas and occult characters, the Franks – from clerics and monks to laypeople – may have thus placed genuine hope and trust in the power of spoken and written words. Whose words these were, and which forces were thought to underly them, is another matter altogether.[13] The tension between Gregory's condemnations and Marcellus' preservation reflects, I suggest, not hypocrisy or inconsistency but different epistemological and social contexts. Monastic medicine could afford ambiguity because monks operated within controlled contexts where intention and framing could be monitored. Monasteries possessed both the literacy to record such practices and the institutional authority to frame them as legitimate Christian medicine.

The Frankish theologian Rabanus Maurus, in the ninth century, reiterated Augustine's condemnation of *praecantationes* and *notae* ("symbols," also called *characteres*).[14] What constituted superstitious use, though? Augustine had argued that efficacy derived from demon intervention rather than textual power, making practitioners' intentions central to legitimacy. But graphophagic remedies typically invoked divine names, biblical verses, and Christian formulae – precisely the authorised content that should work through divine rather than demonic agency. Perhaps the problem was that they mobilised this content through material consumption rather than semantic interpretation, erasing the distinction between spiritual reading and physical eating that theology tried to maintain?

The lack of surviving manuscripts from the Merovingian period, as well as the political and ideological agenda of Carolingian churchmen, are two key elements that must be taken into account. Aside from very isolated cases,[15]

12 E.g.: Paris, BNF, MS Latin 6880, fols. 36r, 42r, 64r, 65r–v, 91v, 92v, 106r, 122v; or the ninth-century northern Italian manuscript Uppsala, Universitetsbiblioteket C. 664, pp. 177ff. On archaeological evidence, see Ildar Garipzanov, "Graphic Ciphers and the Early Medieval Practices of *Collectio* and Concealment," in *Crafting Knowledge in the Early Medieval Book: Practices of Collecting and Concealing in the Latin West*, ed. Sinéad O'Sullivan and Ciaran Arthur (Brepols, 2023), 409–38, at 429–30; Genevra Kornbluth, "Amulets and Identity in the Merovingian World," in *The Oxford Handbook to the Merovingian World*, 941–67.

13 Peregrine Horden, "What's Wrong with Early Medieval Medicine?," *Social History of Medicine* 24, no. 1 (2011): 5–25, at 8.

14 See the aforementioned passage in Augustine's *De doctrina christiana*; Rabanus Maurus, *De institutione clericorum*, ed. Detlev Zimpel, 2 vols. (Brepols, 2006), vol. 2, iii, c. 16, 518.

15 Garipzanov, "Magical Charaktêres."

the typical characters used in Roman Egypt and in late-antique occult practices disappeared in the early medieval West, especially during the Carolingian and Ottonian periods until the twelfth and thirteenth centuries, when they were reimported in Western practices from Byzantine and Islamic sources.[16] However, practices officially banned by Christian bishops persisted and continued to be perceived as effective and valuable resources. Contrary to what Valerie Flint has suggested,[17] what Christian authorities labelled as "magic" was "always there, as a social practice, from the beginning of civilisation through the Greek and Roman world and into the Middle Ages."[18] Magic did not merely exist outside of Christianity to later be Christianised, but it permeated early medieval society at different levels and was "part of society's cultural and social heritage."[19] Some of these practices were, of course, explicitly condemned, but the context remained intrinsically nuanced and fluid. They survived because of a socially accepted belief in their efficacy and, more specifically considering the aims of this book, they were incorporated – at least to a certain extent – into medical practice and religious rituals.

Judging by Isidore of Seville's influential encyclopaedia of the knowledge of his times, Apollo invented the art of medicine, establishing a school founded on the use of *remedia et carmina* ("remedies and charms").[20] The second school was linked to his son Aesculapius, who refined Apollo's teachings by incorporating empirical observation. The third one was associated with Aesculapius' descendant Hippocrates, whose approach relied on logic and rational analysis. This is likely the earliest medieval account of the history of medicine, in which, following Galenic tradition, the author defines medicine as the art that preserves and safeguards bodily health through attention to hygiene and diet.[21] However, Merovingian – and, later, Carolingian – medical

16 Matthew W. Dickie, *Magic and Magicians in the Greco-Roman World* (Routledge, 2001), esp. 304–10; Grévin and Véronèse, "Les 'caractères' magiques"; Richard Gordon, "Charaktêres between Antiquity and Renaissance: Transmission and Re-invention," in *Les savoirs magiques et leur transmission de l'Antiquité à la Renaissance*, ed. Véronique Dasen and Jean-Michel Spieser (SISMEL – Edizioni del Galluzzo, 2014), 253–300; Gideon Bohak, "Jewish Magic in the Middle Ages," in *The Cambridge History of Magic and Witchcraft in the West: From Antiquity to the Present*, ed. David J. Collins (Cambridge University Press, 2015), 268–99.

17 Flint, *The Rise of Magic.*

18 Hen, "The Early Medieval West," 197.

19 Ibid.

20 Isidoro di Siviglia, *Etimologie*, IV, 3–4, 387–8.

21 Pliny the Elder had claimed that medicine came first. Human ambition to improve life, he suggested, allowed magic to insinuate itself – slithering, like a serpent, into human society – presenting itself as a higher, more sacred branch of medicine. It became a form

traditions do not appear to rely on *carmina* and special *characteres* to the same extent as Anglo-Saxon medicine.[22] It can hardly be denied that early medieval continental medical literature was largely composed of classical and late antique texts, often without overtly Christianised content.[23] Gregory of Tours' medical knowledge, as reconstructed by Faith Wallis, drew heavily on Dioscorides' herbal medicine, a longstanding authority for several centuries.[24] Nevertheless, Galenic medicine was also assimilated into "the medicine of Christianity."[25] In other terms, conventional medical practice and miraculous intervention were understood as part of a single cultural framework, rather than as mutually exclusive approaches. Christian miracles, after all, remained an essential – if not the primary – resource. The interconnections between body and soul, and the related sacralisation of medicine, became even more manifest in Carolingian times.[26]

Graphophagy could be sacralised, too. Venantius Fortunatus, bishop of Poitiers, recounts in his hagiography of St. Germanus that a sick monk, bedridden with fever for two years, was healed when he licked an epistle signed by the saint, effectively wiping the signature with his tongue. "Health entered his body, and the ink's inscription proved more powerful than all ointments," reads Venantius' text.[27] An eminent man named Leudegisilus reportedly followed a

---

of medicine that combined "science" with the powers of "religion," sustained by the most alluring promises. Pliny the Elder, *Naturalis Historia*, xxx, 1.1–2. On Isidore's knowledge of Pliny, see for instance Lynn Thorndike, "Some Medieval Conceptions of Magic," *The Monist* 25, no. 1 (1915): 107–139, at 108. When Isidore discusses "magic" specifically, he describes it in purely Augustinian terms. Isidoro di Siviglia, *Etimologie*, viii, 9.3, 700–1. See also Flint, *The Rise of Magic*, 51.

22 Palmer, "Merovingian Medicine," 24–5.

23 Claire Burridge, "Healing Body and Soul in Early Medieval Europe: Medical Remedies with Christian Elements," *Studies in Church History* 58 (2022): 46–67, at 51. See also Ead., *Carolingian Medical Knowledge and Practice, c. 775–990. New Approaches to Recipe Literature* (Brill, 2024).

24 Faith Wallis, "Gregory of Tours' Nosebleed," in *Une traversée des savoirs. Mélanges offerts à Jackie Pigeaud*, ed. Philippe Heuzé, Yves Herant, and Éric Van Der Schueren (Presses de l'Université Laval, 2008), 417–36; Horden, "What's Wrong," 8. See also Rampton, *Trafficking with Demons*, 363–74.

25 Vivian Nutton, "Medicine in Late Antiquity and the Early Middle Ages," in *The Western Medical Tradition: 800 BC to AD 1800*, ed. Laurence I. Conrad, Michael Neve, Vivian Nutton, Roy Porter, and Andrew Wear (Cambridge University Press, 1995), vol. 1, 71–87, at 75. See also Joel L. Gamble, "A Defense of the Carolingian 'Defense of Medicine:' Introduction, Translation, and Notes," *Traditio* 75 (2020): 87–125.

26 Meg Leja, "The Sacred Art: Medicine in the Carolingian Renaissance," *Viator* 47, no. 2 (2016): 1–34.

27 Venantius Fortunatus, *Vita Germani Parisiaci*, ed. Wilhelm Levison, MGH SSRM 7 (Hahn, 1920), lvii, 406–7: "Et quoniam suo merito semina salutis per qua dispersa sunt, contigit,

similar practice whenever someone in his household fell ill with fever or chills: he would wash the letters of Germanus' signature, presumably collecting the water and administering it to the sick.[28]

From the late eighth century onwards, Carolingian reforms encouraged an expansion in manuscript production, including texts of medicine.[29] Recipes appear in a variety of contexts, from manuscripts focused entirely on medical topics to miscellanies containing educational and devotional texts.[30] This variety highlights just how diverse the uses of such texts could be. *Scriptoria* in monastic and cathedral centres were far from isolated workshops; the evidence of multiple scribal hands, glosses, and later additions in medical codices shows that these manuscripts were actively used over generations, serving both as tools for learning and as practical guides for their owners.[31]

Efforts to validate medicine had to face delicate issues, including its pagan origins and the risk of misusing natural ingredients.[32] The *Lorscher Arzneibuch* ("Lorsch Leechbook"), compiled around 800 AD at the German monastery of Lorsch, makes this clear: physicians were keen to defend their knowledge from accusations of impiety, ensuring that medical practice was firmly placed within a Christian framework in order not be dismissed as "magic."[33] At the same time, the ingestion of words and formulae did not *per se* collide with

ut venerabilis Flamiris abba de Canone Toronico manu beati Germani subscriptam accepisset epistolam. Qui cum suum monachum per duos annos febribus decubantem ad lectulum visitaret, requiret infirmus, unde venisset pagina. Respondit abba a domno Germano sibi fuisse directam. Quam petiit sibi porrigi. Qui de subscriptione eius lingua detergens litteram, salus discessit in viscera, et atramenti pictura cuncta vicit unguenta. Unde adprobatum est, languido recuperato, ut dicamus communiter, de sancti subscriptionem sibi sanitatem linxisse." See also Joseph-Claude Poulin, "Entre la magie et la religion. Recherches sur les utilisations marginales de l'écrit dans la culture populaire du haut Moyen Age," in *La culture populaire au Moyen Âge*, ed. Pierre Boglionidir (Les Éditions Univers, 1979), 123–43, at 141.

28 Venantius Fortunatus, *Vita Germani*, xlviii, 402–3: "Leudegisilus inluster, iuxta quod ipse professus est, cum aliquis ex familiae suae domu incurreret typum cuiuscumque aut aliquid frigoris, lavans illas litteras, quas in subscriptionem manus sancta depinxerat, conplures suos hac medella saluti restituit."

29 Vivian Nutton, "Early Medieval Medicine and Natural Science," in *The Cambridge History of Science 2: Medieval Science*, ed. David C. Lindberg and Michael H. Shank (Cambridge University Press, 2013), 323–40.

30 Peregrine Horden, "Sickness and Healing," in *The Cambridge History of Christianity 3: Early Medieval Christianities, c. 600–1100*, ed. Thomas F.X. Noble and Julia M.H. Smith (Cambridge University Press, 2008), 416–32.

31 Burridge, *Carolingian Medical Knowledge*, esp. 19–21.

32 Leja, "The Sacred Art," 5–6.

33 *Medieval Medicine. A Reader*, ed. Faith Wallis (University of Toronto Press, 2010), 84–93. The source is in: *Das 'Lorscher Arzneibuch'. Ein medizinisches Kompendium des 8.*

traditional medicine. As Christian elements were progressively incorporated into medicine during the Carolingian age – which represented "a major break with the classical material"[34] – graphophagic remedies embedded in Christian and socially sanctioned texts continued to be copied and practiced, and thus approved.[35] Whether this persistence was due to their perceived efficacy, their accumulated authority, or both remains an open question.[36]

Starting from the ninth century, special characters and words began to appear with greater frequency, both within the main text and in marginalia. As the Carolingian world transitioned into the ninth and early tenth century, changes in intellectual and institutional contexts – such as the rise of cathedral schools in northern France and renewed theoretical interests in southern Italy – point to new directions in medical learning and writing.[37] Shifts in manuscript production and educational methods suggest that audiences were evolving alongside the uses for medical and recipe literature. In this context, medical writing became part of broader cultural practices of reading, copying and teaching, which ushered in new forms of engagement with graphophagy and the manipulation of texts.[38]

For instance, in a late ninth-century codex – a collection of pastoral text likely copied in north-eastern Francia – a series of characters intended for inscription on parchment (and possibly to be placed on the head) appears in the right-hand margin of one leaf.[39] Similarly, a contemporary manuscript from northern Italy, now preserved in the Abbey Library of Saint Gall, recommends writing the words "emigranius grani. oranio ani. onio ioo. sanat" as a

Jahrhunderts (*Codex Bambergensis medicinalis 1*). *Text, Übersetzung und Fachglossar*, ed. Ulrich Stoll (Franz Steiner, 1992), 48–63.

34 Burridge, "Healing Body and Soul."

35 Meg Leja, *Embodying the Soul: Medicine and Religion in Carolingian Europe* (University of Pennsylvania Press, 2022), 113–6.

36 Rampton, *Trafficking with Demons*, 366–74. Cf. Jolly, *Popular Religion*, 101–3, and Arthur, *"Charms," Liturgies, and Secret Rites*, passim.

37 Claire Burridge, "Early Medieval Recipe Collections: Continuity, Change and the Carolingian Contest," in *Early Medieval Medicine in Context. Transmission, Translation and Transformation*, ed. Debby Banham, Claire Burridge, and Lea T. Olsan (Boydell & Brewer, 2025), 114–63.

38 Katharine Park, "Medicine and Society in Medieval Europe, 500–1500," in *Medicine in Society: Historical Essays*, ed. Andrew Wear (Cambridge University Press, 1992), 59–90, at 66–7; Faith Wallis, "The Experience of the Book: Manuscripts, Texts, and the Role of Epistemology in Early Medieval Medicine," in *Knowledge and the Scholarly Medical Traditions*, ed. Don G. Bates (Cambridge University Press, 1995), 101–26.

39 London, British Library, Add MS 19725, fol. 40r. Cf. Franz Kerff, "Frühmittelalterliche pharmazeutische Rezepte aus dem Kloster Tegernsee," *Sudhoffs Archiv* 67, no. 1 (1983): 111–16, at 115.

remedy for migraine.[40] The words were not intended for ingestion, yet the gradual shortening of the phrases and the loss of consonants hint at a sympathetic logic, aimed at drawing the pain away and making it vanish. In the same folio, a remedy for epistaxis instructs that the phrase "pater talent oli" be written three times on the patient's forehead using the blood dripping from their nose. Another, aimed at relieving "pain in the breasts," prescribes inscribing "filacteria copni" on a laurel leaf.[41] All such formulae consist of both intelligible and uncomprehensible terms. By contrast, spoken words were employed in preparing an antidote for snakebite: as rue was gathered, another series of partly intelligible and partly obscure words were to be recited, and the same formula repeated while the herb was mixed with *aqua pisili* and consumed by the patient.[42]

Graphophagic remedies begin to appear around the same period. A ninth-century collection of medical texts, likely compiled in northern Italy, contains several recipes that reflect this (re)emerging practice. This manuscript is a composite corpus of therapeutic texts that circulated from Late Antiquity into the early Middle Ages. Among its contents is the so-called *Ad cauculum*, a collection of ninety-two recipes in which *praecantationes*, *voces magicae*, and *characteres* play a prominent role.[43] Alongside the more familiar remedies involving *lamellae* inscribed with Greek or other characters, the collection also includes a recipe calling for the recitation of a particular name over a sorrel root, which was then to be chewed to relieve toothache.[44] Another instructs

---

40 St. Gallen, Stiftsbibliothek, Cod. Sang. 44, p. 341. See also *Frühmittelalterliche Rezeptarien*, ed. Julius Jörimann (Orell Fussli, 1925).

41 As observed above, laurel leaves were among the most popular surfaces for written amulets since antiquity. Christopher A. Faraone, *The Transformation of Greek Amulets in Roman Imperial Times* (University of Pennsylvania Press, 2018), 81–2.

42 St. Gallen, Stiftsbibliothek, Cod. Sang. 44, p. 350.

43 On this manuscript, see Arsenio Ferraces Rodríguez, "Magia, medicina y veterinaria en la antigüedad tardía. *Editio princeps* del recetario médico *Ad cauculum*," *Maia* 65, no. 1 (2013): 75–94; Id., "Liber compositionum medicinalium Sangallense-Upsaliensis (= "das St. Galler antidotarium", Sigerist, pp. 78–99)," *Galenos: Rivista di filologia dei testi medici antichi* 15 (2021): 33–58.

44 Uppsala, Universitetsbiblioteket C. 664, p. 178: "Ad dentium dolore*m*. hoc nomen sup*er* scriptum sup*er* *radicem* lapati et coctam dentiu*m* dolore*m* fac*it* ce[s]sare. radix quidem masticata et sup*er* inposita aqua uero coluere sup*er* dicendo nomen summe et bene facit." Sorrel is a lemon-flavoured herb whose cooling properties can provide temporary relief. Its root has long been used in folk medicine for a variety of purposes, notably for its anti-inflammatory and antimicrobial effects. Helena Korpelainen and Maria Pietiläinen, "Sorrel (*Rumex acetosa* L.): Not Only a Weed but a Promising Vegetable and Medicinal Plant," *The Botanical Review* 86 (2020): 234–46, at 239.

writing the same name on galingale leaves (*iuncus triangularis*, a species of *Cyperus*) and chewing them to treat aphthous ulcers in the mouth.[45]

A German *antidotarium* from the late ninth or early tenth century takes things a step further, combining a complex herbal recipe with observations of the sky in a rather unusual fashion. After mixing a selection of herbs and plants with egg whites, the concoction was left for twenty-three days to ferment, during which time worms – probably fly larvae or other insects attracted to the decaying matter – would appear. The fermented mixture, worms included, was then ground and left to mature for another forty days, after which honey was added on top. This preparation was believed to improve the patient's memory.[46] Its efficacy was thought to increase if certain words were recited while tasting it: *alotomentum sedraoton terfice isfinias nereta despone permofinet ment, hec mihi et platoni in usum erat*. As with the formula recorded in Cod. Sang. 44, for gathering rue, this example shows how ordinary words could transform into ritualised vocabulary within such contexts, especially evident in the final section of the formula.[47] The procedure was to be performed during the waxing moon, when it occupied a specific position relative to the zodiac sign Taurus.

Usually, recipes were less elaborate. In a vellum codex compiled during the first half of the century in the Loire region at the monastery of Fulda, which contains Isidore of Seville's *Etymologiae* and inscriptions from the church of the Holy Sepulchre, a few medical recipes were added on the final folio

---

45 Ibidem: "Ad passiones qu*ae* sunt intra os siue rostru*m*. acceptis de decipro foliis tribus sup*er* scribe hoc nom*en* in uno et infusum aceto temperato da ad masticandum. intra unum diem faciet sanu*m* qui ulcera habet." Cypress leaves have been used to treat inflammation, toothache, and laryngitis. Mohd K. Hussain, Mohammad Saquib, Tanveer Ahamad, Shahnaaz Khatoon, and Mohammad Faheem Khan, "Mediterranean Cypress 'Cupressus sempervirens:' A Review on Phytochemical and Pharmacological Properties," *Current Traditional Medicine* 5, no. 4 (2019): 278–97.

46 Bamberg, Staatsbibliothek, MS Med. 2 (L.III.6), fols. 69v–70r. Edition: *Studien und Texte zur Frühmittelalterlichen Rezeptliteratur*, ed. Henry E. Sigerist (Verlag von Johann Ambrosius Barth, 1923), 22–39, here 30: "herba margelli cum uerbascum cacrimonium uiride tritum cum herba fleomon et hibeos et oui albores e quantum deposita diebus uiginti tres fermento nascuntur uermis hos cum supra teres et depone aliis diebus quadraginta et inuenies adhuc eum, hec cum melle misce summo et tere ad memoriam. Est enim potentissimum si per singulos annus cum melle gustis dicens hec: alotomentum sedraoton terfice isfinias nereta despone permofinet ment, hec mihi et platoni in usum erat. Facit autem hec superscripta luna crescentem in decima signo tauri obseruauis his ab omnibus triginta et accipis ut dictum est, sed caue nec aliquem annus intermittam, si non accipiendo et tibi nimie et aspeduculorum nocebit herba quam ipsa est flegmon herba quam mercurius hac illi dedit pro carmina discendat ipsa est quam rustie frusam uocant unde paleam ordeum pellunt."

47 Versnel, "The Poetics of the Magical Charm," 140–1. In this case, the final words have remained understandable, as they read: "this was of help to both me and Plato."

by various hands.[48] Two of these, written by the same scribe at the bottom of the leaf, concern rabies – a disease greatly feared for its potentially fatal consequences.[49] On the left is a remedy for curing a rabid dog, while on the right is one for treating a person bitten by such a dog (fig. 8).

The first remedy, on the left, appears to call for the recitation of an assonant Christian formula over bread – "rabia tabia atq*ue* p*ro* avia. dep*re*cor te ut accipias ..." – accompanied by three Pater Noster, after which the bread was fed to the sick dog. On the right, the same scribe recommends inscribing a more complex formula on bread, combining Christian references with assonant phrases and words. This bread was then given to eat to either afflicted patients or swine exposed to rabies.[50]

Incantations for treating rabid dogs stretched back centuries,[51] and could include the names of deities or other mythological figures. One example is a third-century manuscript written in demotic, closely related to the Greek

48 Leiden, Universiteitsbibliotheek MS VLF 74, fol. 189r. On this manuscript, see Karel A. de Meyier and P.F.J. Obbema, *Codices Vossiani Latini*, Pars I: *Codices in folio* (Universitaire pers Leiden, 1973), 153–5. I'm grateful to Claire Burridge for bringing this and other manuscripts to my attention.

49 Christopher R. Clason, "Animal, Birds, and Fish in the Middle Ages," in *Handbook of Medieval Culture. Volume 1*, ed. Albrecht Classen (de Gruyter, 2015), 18–54, at 42–4.

50 Leiden, Universiteitsbibliotheek MS VLF 74, fol. 189r: "Contra morsu*m* rabiae, sive taccu*m* porcinu*m*. Caput rapit atq*ue* paravit. maxima ripp*ae* atq*ue* petivit. D*eu*s genitoru*m* tuoru*m* + D*eu*s genitoru*m* / meoru*m* + dixit David + Maximeon + capud rabiae + bris colonis tersis + bris conebernis + bris dicto nomine + sic grego ramine + hoc scribe in pane et da manducare cui opus e*st* sive homini *v*el porco." Bread inscribed with words and crosses is similarly a remedy for sick pigs in London, British Library Egerton MS 821, fol. 57v. A spoken blessing on bread was instead recommended to cure porcine dermatitis and, in general, all diseases of cattle, in a ninth-century interpolation to *Medicina Plinii* from the monastery of St. Gallen. St. Gallen, Stiftsbibliothek, 751, p. 441: "Ad morbum porcorum super panem dicas: In nomine Patris et filii et spiritus sancti. Oratione dominica contradicas: agius est, agius est, agius est, sanctus est ille porcus, qui de isto pane manducat nec de thalau nec de purpuriolo nec de nullo morbo morire non debeat; In nomine Patris et filii et spiritus sancti; tertia vice hoc dicas super panem et sic ieiuni porci manducent. Item ad morbum omnium pecurum * chavit rauto + ad qui bany + dep*re*cor te ut maxime retor." See also Geneviève Xhayet, *Médecine et arts divinatoires dans le monde bénédictin médiéval d'après les réceptaires de Saint-Jacques de Liège* (Garnier, 2010), 175–6; Richard Heim, *Incantamenta magica Graeca latina*, Jahrbücher für classische Philologie, suppl. Bd XIX (Teubner, 1893), 563–4. This blessing is almost identical to another one found in London, British Library, Sloane MS 475, f. 114v, a collection of medical texts, prognostics, and more, compiled between the end of the eleventh and the beginning of the twelfth century in Latin, Old French, and Anglo-Norman.

51 Arnaud Tarantola, "Four Thousand Years of Concepts Relating to Rabies in Animals and Humans, Its Prevention and Its Cure," *Tropical Medicine and Infectious Disease* 2, no. 2, 5 (2017), doi: 10.3390/tropicalmed2020005.

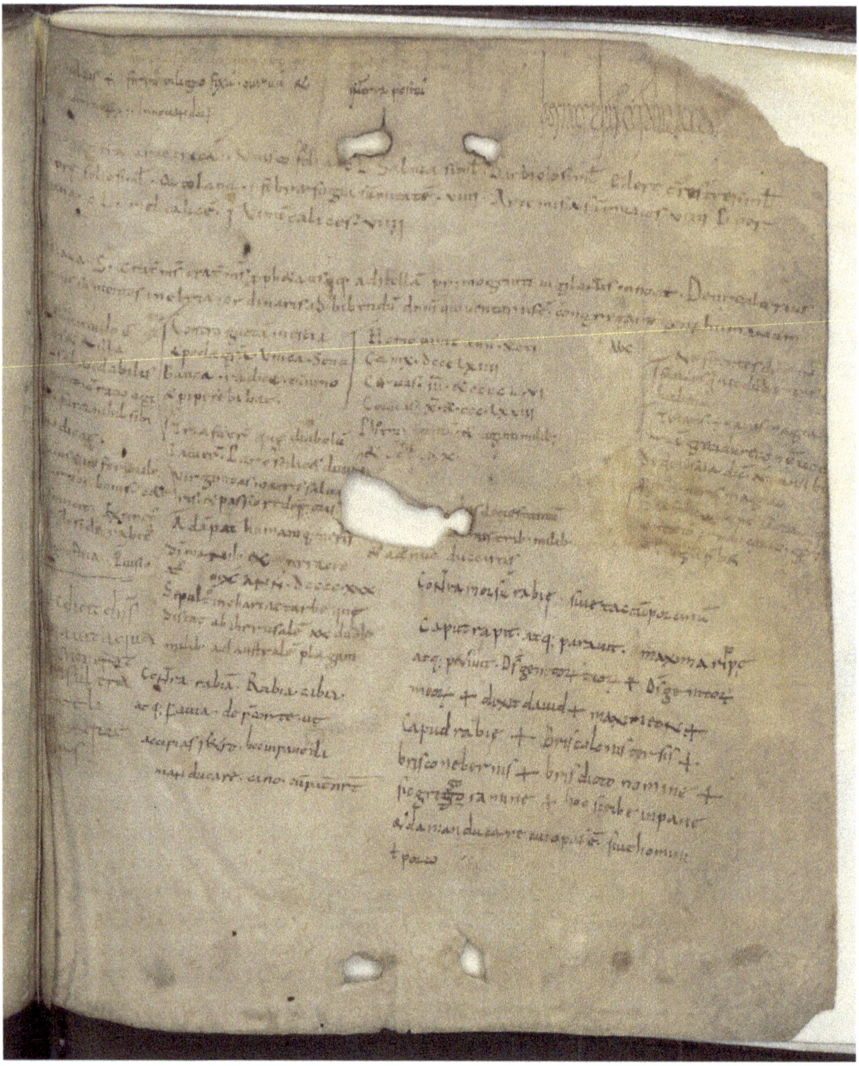

FIGURE 8 Since rabies was considered a dangerous and potentially diabolical disease, its treatment often involved the recitation of Christian prayers alongside the medicinal remedies. Leiden, Universiteitsbibliotheek MS VLF 74, fol. 189r (Source: Leiden University Libraries)

magical papyri from Egypt.[52] It is possible, then, that the obscure or seemingly undecipherable words found in Carolingian remedies for rabies are corrupted versions of names or terms inherited from these late-antique traditions.

52 *The Demotic Magical Papyrus of London and Leiden*, ed. Francis L. Griffith and Herbert Thompson (H. Grevel&Co., 1904), 123–5 and 127.

Dog-bite spells were commonly employed for the most dangerous illnesses – those "from which one can neither recover by oneself nor be healed through medicine."[53] Classical medicine, in turn advanced knowledge of rabies: the fifth-century Graeco-Roman physician Caelius Aurelianus provided a detailed account of its symptoms.[54] Yet charms and special words were not part of the remedies discussed by figures such as Aristotle, Celsus, Dioscorides, Apsyrtos, or Alexander of Tralles. Later, Muslim physicians including al-Rāzī and Ibn Sīna considered treatments for rabies in their writings, but graphophagy does not appear to have been a standard approach whatsoever.[55] Still, material evidence shows that textual remedies could be incorporated into practical treatments: a bowl made in Syria around 1168 for the ruler Nūr al-Dīn Maḥmūd ibn Zangī – the oldest surviving example of its kind – indicates that cures for rabies, among other ailments, could involve inscribed text on bowls, to be diluted with milk, water or oil.[56]

One notes that, within that cultural context, graphophagy was taken into consideration when dealing with several ailments, some of which also emerge in Western sources. In fact, although rabies had been a well-known disease since ancient times, the widespread belief that the illness related to demonic possession in both humans and animals remained popular due to its typical symptoms, among which were restlessness, fury, yelling, feeling of suffocation.[57] Carolingian and post-Carolingian manuscripts prescribe the ingestion

53 Wu Yuhong, "Rabies and Rabid Dogs in Sumerian and Akkadian Literature," *Journal of the American Oriental Society* 121, no. 1 (2001): 32–43, at 32.

54 Jean Théodoridès, "Rabies in Byzantine Medicine," *Dumbarton Oaks Papers, 1984, Vol. 38, Symposium on Byzantine Medicine* (Dumbarton Oaks, 1984), 149–58, at 153–4. See Caelius Aurelianus, *De Morbis Acutis*, 3.9–16; 3.121; 3.132.

55 Bill Wasik and Monica Murphy, *Rabid. A Cultural History of the World's Most Diabolical Virus* (Viking, 2012).

56 Khalili Collection of Islamic Art, Inv. no. MTW1443. The outside of the object features the following text: "This blessed cup is for every poison. In it have been gathered proven uses, and these are for the sting of the serpent, scorpion and fever, for a woman in labour, the abdominal pain of a horse caused by eating earth, and for the bites of a rabid dog, for abdominal pain and colic, for migraine and throbbing pain, for hepatic and splenic fever, for increasing strength, for stopping haemorrhage, for chest pain, for the eye and vision, for driving out spirits, for releasing the bewitched, and for all diseases and afflictions. If one drinks water or oil or milk from it, one will be cured, by the help of the God Almighty." Trans. In Emilie Savage-Smith, "Medicine in Medieval Islam," in *The Cambridge History of Science*, ed. David C. Liindberg, and Michael H. Shank (Cambridge University Press, 2013), 139–67, at 161, fig. 5.3. Nuūr al-Dīn Mahmuūd founded the great hospital of Damascus bearing his name. Although learned physicians never mentioned the use of similar bowls, their existence hint at a certain medical pluralism where elite and popular remedies joined at the seams. Savage-Smith, "Medicine in Medieval Islam," 160–2.

57 Andrea Nicolotti, "A Cure for Rabies or a Remedy for Concupiscence? A Baptism of the Elchasaites," *Journal of Early Christian Studies* 16, no. 4 (2008): 513–34; Nadine Metzger,

of undecipherable words for the same purpose. In a *marginale* of a late tenth- or early eleventh-century manuscript preserved in Trier, a monk recorded a remedy for rabies and the bite of raging quadrupeds which recommends writing the following words on a loaf of bread: "Bis serona +. que + dissipis. Creade +. dettonis +. sicconte + karama+" – in the manuscript, the crosses are placed above the words preceding them.[58] Could there be any link between "bis serona," which appears in this manuscript, and "bris colonis" in the aforementioned codex preserved in Leiden?

Possibly. The same tradition of treating rabies through the repetition of particular forms or sounds (*bis/bris*), and the use of unusual assonant words – whose meaning may or may not have been known by the scribes – appears elsewhere. The words "Bis. groniber sis. bis groniter sis. bis dictoris. sigris grogramini" are featured in a remedy *cui lupus aut canis momorderit*, one of a series of additions made around the year 1000 to a manuscript from Reims (fig. 9).[59]

The words were to be inscribed on the crust of a loaf (possibly incised directly into the dough before baking), although the precise method is not specified here or in any of the other manuscripts. Be that as it may, bread seems to have been a favoured medium for remedies against rabies.

Inscribed bread served other purposes as well, shedding light on another line of continuity between late antiquity and the Early Middle Ages in the practice of graphophagy. These cases reveal the broader circulation of rituals inherited by Christianity. Figures, symbols, letters, names, and phrases had long been used in pagan Europe, and this custom was subsequently incorporated into Christian ritual practice.[60] By late antiquity, people were accustomed to buying bread marked with stamped trademarks or special breads shaped for particular purposes. It was also widely believed that certain breads possessed supernatural powers, as in the Byzantine practice of distributing *hygieia* bread

---

"Kynanthropy: Canine Madness in Byzantine Late Antiquity," *History of Psychiatry* 26, no. 3 (2015): 318–31.

58 Trier, Stadtbibliothek MS 40/1018, fol. 11v. On the manuscript and its marginalia, see Falko Klaes, *Mittelalterliche Glossen und Texte aus Trier. Studien zur volkssprachigen Trierer Überlieferung von den Anfängen bis zum Ende des 11. Jahrhunderts im lateinischen Kontext* (Universitätsverlag Winter, 2017), 321–40. See also Elias von Steinmeyer, ed., *Die kleineren althochdeutschen Sprachdenkmäler* (Weidmann, 1916), 392.

59 Leiden, Universiteitsbibliotheek MS BPL 126, fol. 67v: "Cui lupus aut canis momorderit. hoc scribens in crusta*m* panis da rabiam habenti ad manducand*um*: Bis. groniber sis. bis groniter sis. bis dictoris. sigris grogramini."

60 George Galavaris, *Bread and the liturgy; the symbolism of early Christian and Byzantine bread stamps* (The University of Wisconsin Press, 1970), 22–7.

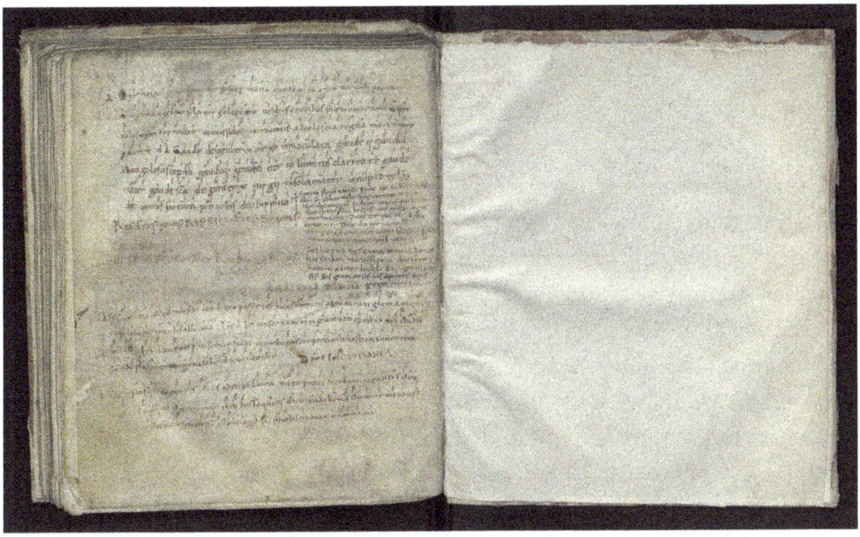

FIGURE 9 Remedies of this kind are often found in *marginalia*, as well as at the beginning or end of manuscripts. Leiden, Universiteitsbibliotheek MS BPL 126, fol. 67v. Leiden University Libraries

to the sick. Bread stamps had been employed for religious purposes since antiquity, and these customs did not undergo radical change over time. Rather, the tradition continued, with symbols and stamps gradually Christianised or adapted to new cultural landscapes. This adaptation, however, did not take place abruptly. For example, before Constantine, when Christians were still persecuted, bread bearing either pagan symbols or disguised Christian ones was preferred.[61] Catechumens received bread of exorcism, a special bread that replaced the Eucharist until they were able to partake.[62] This bread was associated with exorcism because its purpose was to purify the catechumens of evil spirits.

It is not unreasonable to assume that early medieval religious rituals retained elements of pre-Christian practices.[63] One illustrative example is a lesser-known – though no less significant – ordeal: the *iudicium panis et casei*, or ordeal of bread and cheese.[64] This practice was particularly common in the

61 Ibid., 29–31.
62 Ibid., 111.
63 Arthur, *"Charms," Liturgies, and Secret Rites*.
64 Andrea Maraschi and Francesca Tasca, "Aux limites de l'hérésie et de la magie. L'ordalie du pain et du fromage," *Food&History* 16, no. 1 (2018): 49–67.

Frankish-Germanic regions and in England between the tenth and eleventh centuries. In England, it was known as *corsnæd*, where it may have developed in the early eleventh century and was reserved for members of the clergy.[65] More broadly, ordeals served as a last resort, employed when guilt could not be established otherwise.[66]

The *iudicium panis et casei* relied on the invocation of divine judgment, specifically to unmask a thief. Suspects were assembled and required to consume nine *denarii* worth of barley bread (sometimes dry or unleavened) along with an equal amount of hard goat or sheep's cheese.[67] The ordeal's difficulty did not stem from the ritual itself – especially when compared with other ordeals, such as those involving icy water or red-hot iron – but rather from the test it imposed: the guilty were identified as those unable to swallow the consecrated elements. This failure could be attributed both to the physical challenge of chewing and swallowing these hard substances and to the psychological strain of the situation, which would have further hindered the act of swallowing.[68]

The psychological pressure was further intensified by the ritual context. The ordeal elements were first presented on the altar during the celebration of Mass, and they could bear inscriptions believed to possess extralinguistic power. The *Pater Noster* was often written on the bread's crust, while the crust of the cheese might bear the inscription of Psalm 7:17: "Convertetur dolor eius in caput eius, et in verticem eius iniquitas eius descendet" ("The trouble they cause recoils on them; their violence comes down on their own heads").[69]

A small document (*breviculus*) listing the names of the suspects was prepared and placed on the altar between the bread and cheese. After Mass, the

65 John D. Niles, "Trial by Ordeal in Anglo-Saxon England: What's the Problem with Barley?," in *Early Medieval Studies in Memory of Patrick Wormald*, ed. Stephen Baxter, Catherine Karkov, Janet L. Nelson, and David Pelteret (Routledge, 2009), 369–82.

66 On ordeals, see Patrick Wormald, *Papers Preparatory to the Making of English Law: King Alfred to the Twelfth Century*, vol. 2 (University of London, 2014), 72–90; Peter Browe, *De ordaliis*, 2 vols. (Apud aedes Pont. Universitatis Gregorianae, 1932); Jean Gaudemet, "Les ordalies au Moyen Âge: doctrine, législation et pratique canoniques," in Id., *La société ecclésiastique dans l'occident médiéval* (Variorum Reprints, 1980), 99–135; Bruno Lemesle, ed., *La preuve en justice: de l'Antiquité à nos jours* (Presses universitaires de Rennes, 2003); Peter Brown, "Society and the Supernatural: A Medieval Change," *Daedalus* 104, no. 2 (1975): 133–51.

67 *Ordines iudiciorum Dei*, in Formulae *Merowingici et Karolini aevi. Ordines iudiciorum Dei*, ed. Karl Zeumer (Hahn, 1886), 599–722, at 635.

68 Sarah Larratt Keefer, "*Ut in omnibus honorificetur Deus*: The *corsnæd* Ordeal in Anglo-Saxon England," in *The Community, the Family and the Saint. Patterns of Power in Early Medieval Europe*, ed Joyce M. Hill and Mary Swan (Brill, 1998), 237–64.

69 For instance, *Ordines iudiciorum Dei*, 631 and 635.

priest would recite a ritual formula, invoking biblical scenes in which God vindicates the innocent who have been wrongly accused, such as Susanna in Daniel 13. On occasion, the priest would even address the bread directly, calling for divine judgment to reveal the thief and drawing analogies to biblical events. For example, in reference to the pillar of fire and cloud that prevented the Egyptians from crossing the Red Sea as they pursued the fleeing Israelites (Ex 14:24–25), the priest might invoke the Lord to obstruct the throat of the guilty party, preventing them from swallowing the consecrated elements.

The significance of this act of inscription – which was then transformed into graphophagy – must have been considerable in a world in which divine judgment was unquestioned and analogical thinking was pervasive.[70] As in the *sotah* ritual, graphophagy is not metaphorical but concrete; text is consumed to determine guilt through bodily effects. Moreover, the practice was ancient and carried an inherent authority.[71] Indeed, a non-Christian bread and cheese trial existed at least five or six centuries earlier, if not more, appearing in the *Greek Magical Papyri*. In one formula for unmasking thieves, Greek deities such as Hermes, Helios, Themis, and the Erinyes are invoked alongside Egyptian deities like Ammon and Parammon (the counterparts of Zeus and Hermes).[72] Each deity carried specific symbolic significance: Hermes as the god of thieves, Helios as the sun revealing hidden truths, Themis as the embodiment of law and justice, and the Erinyes as avengers. These deities were called upon to seal the throat of the guilty party, in a striking parallel to the later Christian invocation of the pillar of fire.

The invocation was accompanied by a purification rite, after which the suspects were required to consume a piece of winter wheat bread and goat cheese, each weighing eight drachmas. A fourth-century CE papyrus from Egypt (Berlin, Ägyptisches Museum, P. 17202) contains a similar ritual for unmasking a thief.[73] Although linked to a Christian cultural context, the

70 Robert A. Yelle, "Rhetorics of Law and Ritual: A Semiotic Comparison of the Law of Talion and Sympathetic Magic," *Journal of the American Academy of Religion* 69, no. 3 (2001): 627–48.

71 Danuta Shanzer, "Food of Judgement: Late Antiquity and the Early Middle Ages," in *Early Christian Mystagogy and the Body*, ed. Nienke Vos and Paul van Geest (Peeters, 2022), 467–98, at 488–9. For later cases, see Chiara Benati, "Painted Eyes, Magical Sieves and Carved Runes: Charms for Catching and Punishing Thieves in the Medieval and Early Modern Germanic Tradition," in *Magic and Magicians in the Middle Ages and the Early Modern Time. The Occult in Pre-modern Sciences, Medicine, Literature, Religion, and Astrology*, ed. Albrecht Classen (de Gruyter, 2017), 149–218.

72 PGM V. 172–212.

73 William Brashear and Roy Kotansky, "A New Magical Formulary," in *Magic and Ritual in the Ancient World*, 3–24; Theodore S. de Bruyn and Jitse H.F. Dijkstra, "Greek Amulets

papyrus contains six remedies written in Greek, consistent with rituals found the *Greek Magical Papyri*. The fourth remedy aims to identify the perpetrator of a theft and appears to be a later derivation of the bread and cheese formula found in the aforesaid papyri. Unlike the medieval version, this iteration was likely intended for domestic rather than liturgical use.[74]

None of these late antique bread-and-cheese formulas implied an act of graphophagy. By the fifth century, however, the ritual use of bread and cheese as instruments for unmasking a thief appears to have been not only well established but also practiced in contexts extending beyond than the strictly domestic. This is also suggested by a reference from the Second Council of Ephesus (449), where the Syrian bishop Sophronius of Tella was accused, among other things, of practicing magical arts and participating in "demonic banquets." Among the charges, one specifically alleged that Sophronius conducted divinatory rituals using bread and cheese, together with water, oil, and eggs:

> One day, while Sophronius was traveling, he lost some gold and suspected certain acquaintances of stealing it. Dissatisfied with merely making them swear on the Gospel, he sought to subject them – like pagans – to the ordeal of bread and cheese, forcing them to eat them; yet he did not recover his gold. He then prepared a potion and asked: "Who has my gold? What is their name? What are they wearing?" The demons, undoubtedly eager to deceive him, identified a thief – not out of a desire to punish him but to lead the bishop into perdition.[75]

---

and Formularies from Egypt Containing Christian Elements: A Checklist of Papyri, Parchments, Ostraka, and Tablets," *The Bulletin of the American Society of Papyrologists* 48 (2011): 163–216, at 184, n. 7; David Jordan, "Phallus or Fleas at Berol inv. 17202.31?," *Zeitschrift für Papyrologie und Epigraphik* 141 (2002): 139–41.

74 Rudolf Köstler held that the *iudicium offae* originated in the domestic context of Christian *domus*. Rudolf Köstler, "Der Anteil des Christentums an der Ordalien," *Zeitschrift der Savigny-Stiftung für Rechtsgeschichte: Kanonistische Abteilung* 32, 2 (1912): 208–48, at 242–3.

75 Jean-Pierre Paulin Martin, *Actes du Brigandage d'Ephèse. Traduction faite sur le texte syriaque contenu dans le manuscript 14530 du Musée britannique* (E. Glorieux, 1874), 89–94, at 91. See also: Maijastina Kahlos, "*Artis heu magicis*: The Lable of Magic in Fourth-Century Conflicts and Disputes," in *Pagans and Christians in Late Antique Rome. Conflict, Competition, and Coexistence in the Fourth Century*, ed. Michele Renee Salzman, Marianne Sághy and Rita Lizzi Testa (Cambridge University Press, 2016), 162–177, at 169. The original Greek accusation against Sophronius has been lost, with only a Syriac translation surviving. See also Ernest Honigmann, "A Trial for Sorcery on August 22, A.D. 449," *Isis* 35, no. 4 (1944): 281–3; Silvia Acerbi, "Acusaciones de magia contra obispos: el caso de Sofrino de Tella," *Codex Aquilarensis. Cuadernos de investigación del Monasterio de Santa María la Real* 17 (2001): 129–42, at 139.

Since the ordeal yielded no results, Sophronius resorted to bowl divination: he placed a child before a bowl containing oil and water and, after reciting some incantations, asked the youth to tell him what he was seeing in the bowl.[76]

The ordeal of bread and cheese thus remained, in the fifth century, associated with pagan divinatory practices involving contact with demonic entities. This account underscores both the persistence of such practices and the tensions they generated within Christian religious frameworks. It also shows that some Christian clerics actively contributed to preserving practices originating from late antique pagan and Hermetic traditions, even when these were formally condemned.[77]

These crucial precedents, while they do not involve graphophagy in the way seen in later Christian practice, attest to its non-Christian origins. They demonstrate the Christianisation of a pre-existing mode of thought and associated techniques, which continued to be regarded as legitimate and effective. It is perhaps no coincidence that when Giovanni Boccaccio included a tale centred on the bread and cheese ordeal in the *Decameron*, he used the term *incantagione* ("enchantment") to describe the invocation formula recited over pieces of gingerbread.[78] Moreover, Boccaccio omits any priestly involvement; instead, the tale presents a judicial rite conducted among laypeople in a rural, popular context. The protagonists are the hapless Calandrino and the cunning Bruno and Buffalmacco.

Adolf Jacoby interpreted the act of graphophagy in the context of the *iudicium panis et casei* as magic, citing several analogous practices in other cultures.[79] There is, however, no clear evidence that ordeals in general were widespread in early medieval Europe. Actually, aside from the ordeal of hot water, there is no trace of ordeals as a whole until the eighth century, when the Church seems to have actively promoted their wider use.[80] Robert Bartlett argues that ordeals were primarily Frankish rather than pan-Germanic, as reflected in the Salic law (ca. 510), while a parallel tradition had emerged in

76 Sophronius also practiced φιαλομαντεία or λεκανομαντειᾶ. See Dickie, *Magic and Magicians*, 267.

77 Andrey Yu Vinogradov and Mikhail S. Zheltov, "The 'Apocryphal' Inscription from Mangup, Crimea, and Rituals of 'Exposing the Thief:' Magic and Law from Antiquity to the Middle Ages," *Slověne* 1 (2015): 53–93.

78 Giovanni Boccaccio, *Decameron*, ed. Vittore Branca, 2 vols. (Mondadori, 2005 [1985]), vol. 1, viii, n. 6, 671.

79 Adolf Jacoby, "Der Ursprung des Judicium offae," *Archiv für Religionswissenschaft* 13 (1910): 526–66, at 529: "Wir stehen damit in der Magie drinnen."

80 Henry C. Lea, *The Ordeal* (University of Pennsylvania Press, 1973 [1866]), 30; Robert Bartlett, *Trial by Fire and Water. The Medieval Judicial Ordeal* (Clarendon Press, 1986), 4.

Ireland as early as the seventh century.[81] He further notes that "Frankish influence on Anglo-Saxon ordeals" in the tenth and eleventh centuries "is quite certain."[82] The Carolingians were particularly eager to employ these judicial instruments, drawing on local custom and with the "modelling of new forms on old."[83] Despite being eventually Christianised, however, the ordeal itself was not inherently Christian.

The ordeal of bread and cheese was already practised in England prior to the Norman conquest. According to Sarah Keefer, only a single continental liturgical source – the eleventh-century *Cracow Pontifical* – mentions this rite. By contrast, eight different versions are recorded in English liturgical books.[84] This suggests that the ritual may have originated in the Anglo-Saxon period, before subsequently circulating.[85] Indeed, *corsnæd* is referenced in the *Canons of Edgar*, a legal text drafted by Wulfstan sometime after the reign of King Edgar the Peaceable (959–975). Graphophagy was also a component of this ordeal, indicating that the practice of inscribing the bread and/or cheese must have been introduced at some point – whether in the continent or in England – since it had become culturally and socially acceptable, even within a Christian framework.[86]

In the meantime, the practice of inscribing prayers and biblical verses on specially prepared writing surfaces must have gained full legitimacy in the eyes of clerics. This can also be seen on the upper margin of a tenth-century manuscript of (Pseudo-)Boethius' *Commentaria in Topica Ciceronis* (fig. 10), where the compiler annotated: "Ad furtu*m* inveniuendu*m*. In pane subcinerio scribe et da comedere reo. AKPICA. KPOKA. PICKAPIT. APICAPIT."[87]

The gibberish may be interpreted as an instance of *verba mystica*, or non-semantic formulae typical in protective, diagnostic, or coercive charms, in which verbal symmetry was thought to mirror or enforce cosmic order. The heavy use of certain letters (k, p, i) together with the alternating consonant-vowel rhythm, strongly recalls the graphic and acoustic impression of Greek.

81 Bartlett, *Trial by Fire and Water*, 4–5.

82 Ibid., 7. See also Gustav Glotz, *L'Ordalie dans la Grèce primitive : Étude de droit et de mythologie* (Fontemoing, 1904), 110–1.

83 Bartlett, *Trial by Fire and Water*, 11.

84 Keefer, "*Ut in omnibus honorificetur Deus*," 246.

85 Niles, "Trial by Ordeal in Anglo-Saxon England," 373.

86 As per Cambridge, Corpus Christi College, MS 391, cited in Keefer, "*Ut in omnibus honorificetur Deus*," 262: "adportetur caseus et panis hordeatius et inscribatur in eo oratio dominica …".

87 Cologne, Erzbischöfliche Diözesan- und Dombibliothek, Cod. 198, fol. 76r: "To discover a theft. Write [this] on bread baked under ashes and give it to the accused to eat. AKPICA. KPOKA. PICKAPIT. APICAPIT."

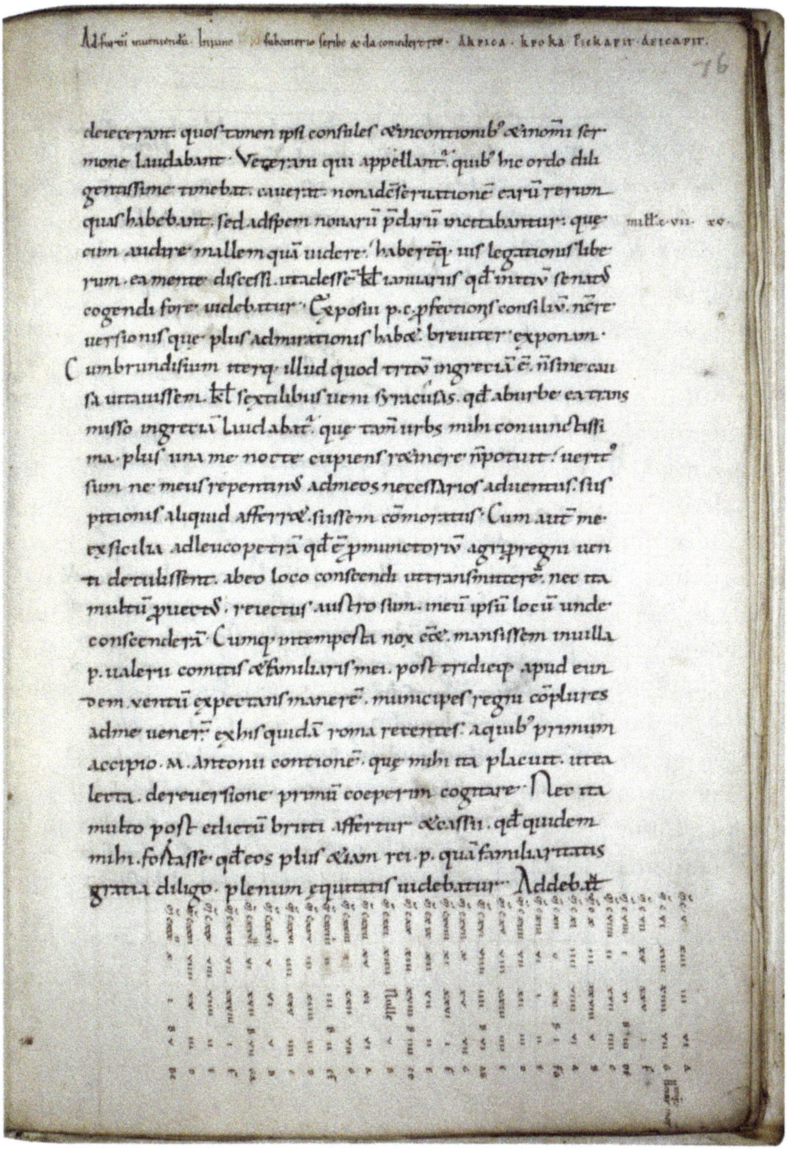

FIGURE 10 A ready-for-use remedy to identify a thief, noted by the compiler in the upper margin of a manuscript, Cologne, Erzbischöfliche Diözesan- und Dombibliothek, Cod. 198, fol. 76r. Reproduced with permission of Erzbischöfliche Diözesan- und Dombibliothek

This is not surprising, given the origins of similar remedies: Greek letters or Greek-like strings functioned as markers of authority, antiquity, and arcane knowledge. It is also worth noting that bread baked under ashes used to be associated with penitential contexts: the *Pontificale Romano-Germanicum*, written between 950 and 962, assigned this specific type of bread to those who were possessed by the devil and were required to observe a severe fast.[88]

There are further elements to consider, though. A suggestive hint comes from a scholium on Horace's *Epistles*, traditionally attributed to the grammarian Helenius Acro (or Acron), who flourished in the second century. The commentary, however, is not the work of Acro himself. Although the attribution to the Roman grammarian became widespread in printed editions, modern scholarship refers to the author as Pseudo-Acro.[89] The incorporation of this scholium into the manuscript tradition may have occurred at various points between classical antiquity, late antiquity, and the early Middle Ages, reflecting a complex history of transmission.

In the epistle in question, Horace writes to his friend Aristius Fuscus that, while the latter preferred life in the city, he himself favoured the countryside. He presents himself as weary of urban comforts, likening his condition to that of a priest's slave who, tired of consuming sacrificial sweets, yearned for simple bread.[90] In the accompanying scholium, Pseudo-Acro explains that the priests' slaves were accustomed to eating large quantities of sacrificial confections.[91] Interestingly, he then adds that when slaves were suspected of theft, they were brought before a priest who administered bread over which he had recited a *carmen*. The guilty party, according to this account, was identified by an inability to swallow the morsel.

> [Acr.] Hor. epist. 1.10.10: cum in servis suspicio furti habetur, ducunt ad sacerdotem, qui crustum panis carmine infectum dat singulis; quod cum h<a>eserit manifestum furti reum asserit.[92]

It would therefore be reasonable to assume that this second observation was added at a later stage, possibly in the ninth century.[93] This testimony

88 *Le Pontifical romano-germanique*, ii, 220–1.

89 Roberto Fiori, "Ordalie e diritto romano," *IURA. Rivista Internazionale di Diritto Romano e Antico* 65 (2017): 1–128, at 70–2.

90 Horace, *Epistles. Book I*, ed. Roland Mayer (Cambridge University Press, 1994), i.10.9–10, 69: "utque sacerdotis fugitivus liba recuso; / pane egeo iam mellitis potiore placentis."

91 *Pseudacronis scholia in Horatium vetustiora*, ed. Otto Keller, 2 vols. (Teubner, 1902–04), ii, 242: "quia sacerdotum servi comedunt multa liba de sacris."

92 Ibidem: "When slaves are suspected of theft, they are brought before a priest who gives each of them a piece of bread imbued with a charm. If it becomes stuck, the priest declares the guilty party of the theft."

93 Fiori, "Ordalie e diritto romano," 72.

is of particular interest, as it occupies a chronological position between the attestations from Graeco-Roman Egypt and the case of Sophronius of Tella on the one hand, and the later proliferation of Carolingian and Anglo-Saxon sources on the other. Although it does not yet involve an act of graphophagy – which thus appears to be a later development – it already articulates the idea that the elements of the ordeal were imbued with the extralinguistic power of specialised words.

From the perspective of the archaeological record, a recent discovery in the basilica of Mangup in Crimea has brought to light a bread stamp dating from the tenth to the twelfth century (thickness: 3.5; diameter: 11.2), engraved with a biblical verse: the first half of Psalm 9:28: "Οὖ ἀρᾶς τὸ στόμα αὐτοῦ γέμη κ(αὶ) πικρίας κὲ δόλου" ("Whose mouth is full of cursing, and bitterness, and fraud") (fig. 11).[94] This artefact seems to be connected to the incantatory formulas for identifying thieves found in the Egyptian papyri and provides further evidence that later Christianised versions of such procedures – also widespread in the Byzantine sphere – were rooted in earlier traditions.

Though the ordeal of bread and cheese was officially prohibited in Constantinople and in the central regions of the Empire during the medieval period, the discovery of this stamp suggests that the practice persisted in peripheral areas. It also reflects the syncretic character of Byzantine rites for identifying thieves, in which Christian elements seem to veil a practice that was fundamentally non-Christian in origin.[95]

The continuity of this ordeal-based practice, in new forms that nonetheless confirm its enduring popularity and authority, is attested in manuscript Egerton 821, now preserved in the British Library. This manuscript is a compendium of texts on astrology, divination, and remedies employing herbs, talismans and charms. It dates to the final quarter of the twelfth century and was compiled in southern France, possibly in the region of Béziers (fig. 12).[96] Notably, it contains a ritual designed to identify the perpetrator of a theft, to which the compiler explicitly draws the reader's attention by means of a *manicula*: "scribe in tribus foliis lauri et voca ad manducandum eum quem

94 This verse does not appear anywhere else in Byzantine epigraphy. See: https://iospe.kcl.ac.uk/5.194.html.

95 Vinogradov and Zheltov, "The 'Apocryphal' Inscription from Mangup."

96 On this city and its cultural context at the time, see Charles Burnett, "Béziers as an Astronomical Center for Jews and Christians in the Mid-Twelfth Century," *Aleph* 17, no. 2 (2017): 197–219.

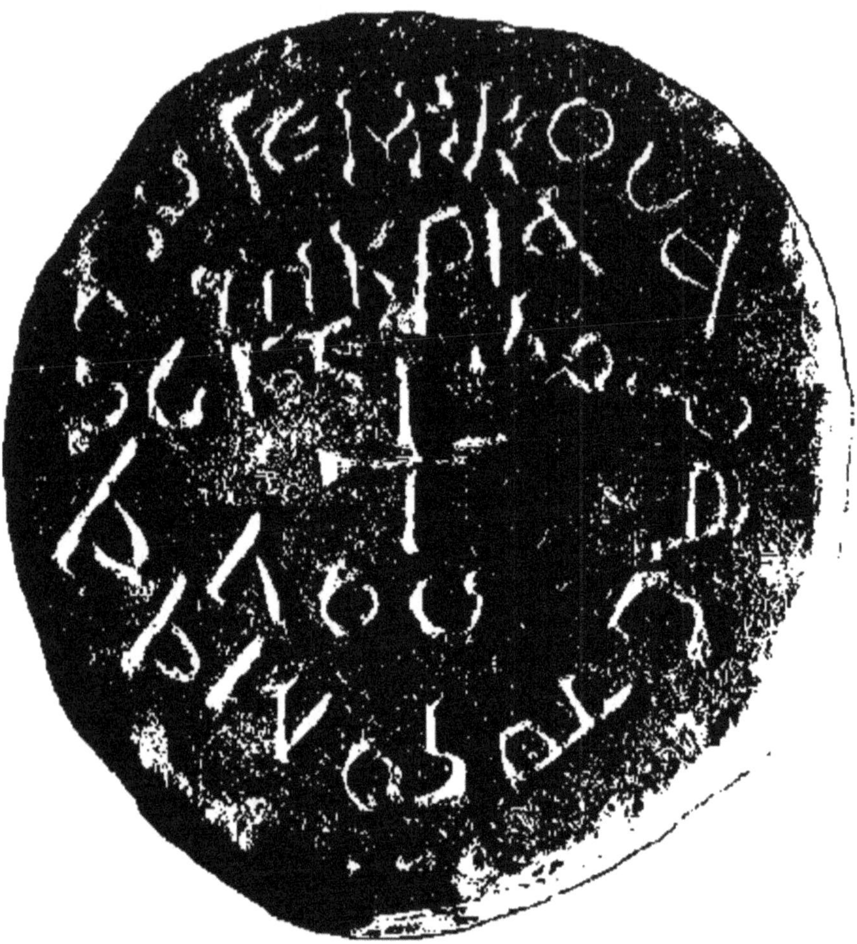

FIGURE 11 Stamp with liturgical inscription used to inscribe the formula on a special bread, found in modern Sevastopol, Crimea. National Preserve of Tauric Chersonesos, n. 11/37269. © 2015 Andrey Vinogradov (edition), Irene Polinskaya (translation)

suspicaris. Et mitte hos caracteres subtus [subter] vas in quo cibus est et non poterit comedere: a.a.d.a.a.i. [symbol] B.a.h."[97]

The aim remains the same, but the means differ. Letters and symbols are to be inscribed on three bay leaves, which are then placed – presumably in secret – beneath the cutting board or platter from which the suspect will

97 London, British Library Egerton MS 821, fol. 34r: "Write on three laurel leaves and summon the suspect to eat. Place these characters beneath the vessel containing the food, and they will be unable to eat: a.a.d.a.a.i. [symbol] B.a.h."

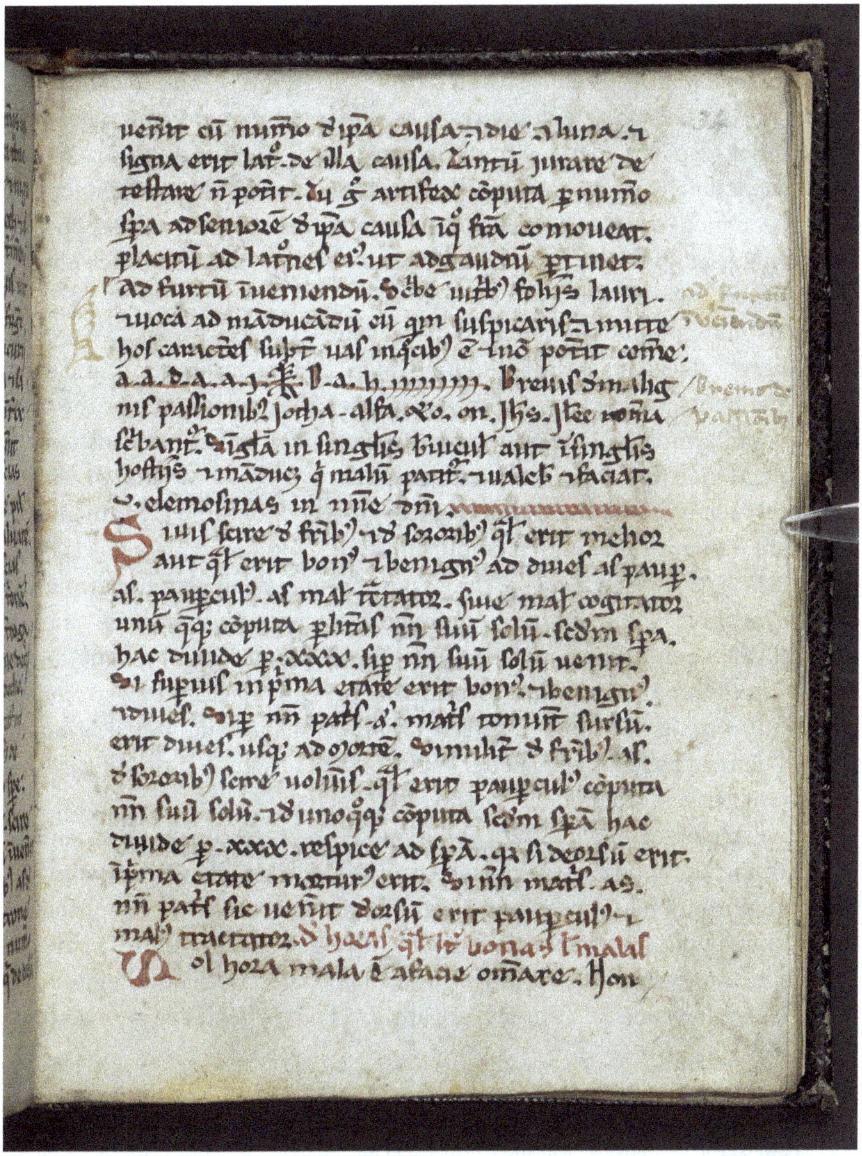

FIGURE 12 The scribe draws the reader's attention to his graphophagic formula to identify a thief. London, British Library Egerton MS 821, fol. 34r. The British Library, Polonsky Pre-1200 Project

take their food. The power of the characters is thereby transferred to the suspect, who becomes unable to swallow even a single morsel. The letters may represent abbreviations or transliterations of Hebrew words, as is the case elsewhere in the same manuscript;[98] for instance, "a" might stand for *Adonai* (God) or *Adam*. One notes the predominance of the letter "a" and the symmetrical arrangement of "d" and "i", which could be read as *adonai adonai dominus adonai adonai iesus*, or alternatively as *agios agios domine agios agios iesu*. The symbol – possibly derived from Greek or Arabic textual traditions – may have functioned as a seal, narking the transition from the invocatory portion of the sequence (the first section) to its coercive component (the second).[99] The recipe itself, however, offers no explanation of the source or mechanism of its efficacy.

Letters and graphic symbols were thus believed to exert their effect even when merely placed in contact with food intended for consumption, and even when that contact was mediated by a container. This reflects one of the core principles of sympathetic logic as reconstructed – correctly, in this instance – by Frazer. At the same time, letters and symbols could prove problematic within a cultural milieu in which Augustine's theory of signs continued to provide the dominant framework for understanding magic.[100] For Augustine, signs (*signa*) were not neutral instruments. While conventional signs could legitimately convey meaning within human communication, non-conventional ones – especially those employed outside liturgical or scriptural contexts – functioned as a means to communicate with demons and perform magic; they were consequently to be condemned. In this sense, what Augustine condemned as *magia* was not defined by technique alone, but by misuse of signs whose efficacy was thought to derive from hidden, non-divine agencies.

This suspicion extended to abbreviations, ciphers, symbols, and talismans alike, all of which appeared to operate beyond intelligible linguistic meaning.[101] From Augustine's perspective, such signs were dangerous precisely because they claimed efficacy without transparent reference to God. In his *De civitate Dei*, while discussing miracles, the Bishop of Hippo describes how demons are invoked and persuaded: "[demons] are attracted not by food like animals, but,

98 For instance, ibid., fol. 59v.

99 On symbols drawn from Greek and Arabic texts, see Nicolas Weill-Parot, "Imprinting Powers: The Astrological Seal and Its Doctrinal Meanings in the Latin West," *The Medieval Globe* 4, no. 1 (2018): 49–72.

100 Robert A. Markus, "Signs, communication and communities in Augustine's *De doctrina christiana*," in De doctrina Christiana: *A Classic of Western Culture*, ed. Duane W.H. Arnold and Pamela Bright (University of Notre Dame Press, 1995), 97–108; Claire Fanger, "For Magic: Against Method," in *The Routledge History of Medieval Magic*, 26–36; Ead., "Magic," in *The Oxford Guide to the Historical Reception of Augustine*, ed. Karla Pollman and Willemien Otten, 3 vols. (Oxford University Press, 2013), vol. 3, 860–5.

101 Benedek Láng, "Characters and Magic Signs in the *Picatrix* and Other Medieval Magic Texts," *Acta Classica Universitatis Scientiarum Debreceniensis* 47 (2011): 69–77.

like spirits, by such symbols [*signa*] as suit their taste, various kinds of stones, woods, plants, animals, songs [*carmina*], rites."[102] It was clear, anyhow, that practicing magic entailed "trafficking" with demons.[103]

The issue became particularly acute from the eleventh and twelfth centuries onwards, when a substantial influx of Greek and Arabic texts entered Western Europe, bringing with them new symbolic systems and ritual technologies that challenged established Christian semiotics. Meanwhile, in Western monastic milieux, manuscripts proliferated in which amulets intended to be carried on the body were accompanied – sometimes explicitly, sometimes more discreetly – by prescriptions for ingesting written texts. In a German miscellany of medicine, astronomy, and mathematics dating from the twelfth century, a meticulously precise remedy for epilepsy instructs that a passage from Mt 4 be written on a wooden tablet "with some kind of black pigment that can be easily washed off." As soon as the patient showed signs of an impending epileptic seizure, the writing was to be washed into a vessel of water and administered for drinking "in the name of the Father, the Son, and the Holy Spirit."[104]

In a roughly contemporary vellum manuscript from Germany, a more elaborate version of the same remedy specifies that the ink should be made from ground charcoal. Here, however, the whole procedure is embedded in a dense framework of Christian ritual practices: the patient was to fast for three days, attend Mass, and the tablet was to be washed in water that had been blessed with exorcised salt. In addition, the patient was instructed to eat bread prepared using the same water.[105]

If the question is whether graphophagy was actively practiced in the Merovingian, Carolingian, and post-Carolingian worlds, the available evidence

102 Agostino, *La città di Dio*, ed. Luigi Alici (Bompiani, 2001), xxi.6.2, 1072.

103 Rampton, *Trafficking with Demons*, 27–8.

104 Paris, BNF, MS Latin 229, f. 7v: "Ante hora*m* accessionis scribe cont*ra* caducum morbum evangeliu*m* sec*un*d*um* math*eum* duct*us* e*st* ies*us* i*n* desertu*m* a sp*iritum* *us*q*ue* angeli accesser*int* et m*isericordia* ei in tabula lignea cu*m* aliqua nig*re*dine que*m* facile ablui possit et mox ut videris egro morbu*m* accedere lavabis scriptura in vas aliq*uo*d cu*m* silenti fonte sic*ut* p*ri*a dixi et dabis ei bib*ere* i*n* no*min*e patris et filii et sp*iritus* *sancti*."

105 Herten, Bibliothek des Grafen Nesselrode-Reichenstein, MS 192. The manuscript was destroyed during the Second World War, but it has been edited in: Karl Sudhoff, "Codex medicus Hertensis (Nr. 192). Handschriftstudie," *Archiv für Geschichte der Medizin* 10, no. 6 (1917): 265–313, here at 301: "Qui caducum morbum patitur debet ienunare tres dies in nomine patris et filii et spiritus sancti et per ipsos tres dies debet audire missam que cantatur pro infirmis et euangelium ductus est iesus in desertum. ipsum scribatur in lignea tabula cum attritis carbonibus et legatur infra missam super capud eius et post lectum euangelium diluatur tubula cum aqua que cum maiori exorcismo salis sit benedicta. et panis quem manducat efficiatur ex ipsa aqua. ipsamque aquam bibat …"

suggests that reliance on the power of spoken and written words began to spread from the ninth century onwards. This period also marks the growing popularity of the *iudicium panis et casei*, now augmented by the inscription of psalms and prayers on the ritual elements. It is hard to determine which side of the English Channel exerted the stronger influence, yet it is worth emphasising the originality of this development, given that earlier forms of the ordeal did not involve the inscription of formulae on bread and cheese. By this point, anyhow, belief in the extralinguistic power of words had once again become sufficiently widespread to surface in a variety of sources, after seemingly receding for a few centuries.

Medical knowledge circulated actively in Merovingian monasteries and episcopal contexts, but it was organised, recorded, and transmitted differently than in Anglo-Saxon England. This hypothesis finds support in the distribution of evidence. Some of the few attestations of graphophagy appear not in formal medical treatises but in *marginalia*, final manuscript folios, and the likes. Graphophagy's relative invisibility in Carolingian medical manuscripts tells us less about practice than about genre, though: such remedies were recorded elsewhere (liturgical ordeal texts) or not recorded formally at all (*marginalia*, oral transmission, local practice). The later Carolingian and post-Carolingian evidence supports this interpretation. By the tenth century, graphophagic remedies appear more frequently in medical manuscripts, reflecting broader changes in the intellectual climate and developments in medical knowledge.[106] Graphophagy probably circulated throughout the early medieval period but achieved manuscript visibility only as textual practices became more accommodating toward remedies lacking classical pedigrees.

106 Burridge, "Healing Body and Soul."

CHAPTER 4

Runes and the Power of Words in Scandinavia

Unlike the contiguous manuscript traditions of Latin Christendom, Viking-Age and medieval Scandinavia operated across a spectrum of literacies that combined runic epigraphy, oral verse, and later manuscript production in Latin. The earliest evidence of literacy in Scandinavia is preserved in the runic corpus, which functioned both as a memorial and communicative script.[1] Parallel to runic practice was the oral tradition of vernacular poetry and saga narrative. Eddic and skaldic verse, while primarily composed and transmitted orally in their early phases, were eventually fixed in manuscript form, most notably in medieval Icelandic codices years after the conversion to Christianity.[2] Here, the bishoprics of Skálholt and Hólar were founded respectively in 1056 and 1106, and became important centres of learning.[3] The later preservation of these poetic corpora reflects a broader process of institutionalisation of vernacular textuality. By the thirteenth century, the production of texts in vernacular Icelandic had grown into a substantial cultural endeavour, marking the flourishing period of saga composition. Despite surviving in manuscripts dating from the thirteenth century onward, sagas represent traditions of composition and performance that significantly pre-date their extant copies.[4]

Medieval Scandinavian written culture was characterised by interactions between oral and literate practices, rather than a simple transition from speech to script.[5] Runes and oral verse intersected with the emergent manuscript culture in ways that shaped the material and medial qualities of texts – an intersection that is crucial to understanding how phenomena such as graphophagy

1 Terje Spurkland, "Literacy and 'runacy' in medieval Scandinavia," in *Scandinavia and Europe 800–1350: Contact, Conflict, and Coexistence*, ed. Jonathan Adams and Katherine Holman (Brepols, 2004), 333–44.

2 Emily Lethbridge, "Manuscripts and Textual Culture," in *The Cambridge History of Old Norse-Icelandic Literature*, ed. Heather O'Donoghue and Eleanor Parker (Cambridge University Press, 2024), 33–49.

3 Ryder Patzuk-Russell, *The Development of Education in Medieval Iceland* (de Gruyter, 2021).

4 Fulvio Ferrari, *Le saghe nordiche. Eroi, vichinghi e poeti nella Scandinavia medievale* (Meltemi, 2022), 43–5.

5 Judy Quinn, "From Orality to Literacy in Medieval Iceland," in *Old Icelandic Literature and Society*, ed. Margaret Clunies Ross (Cambridge University Press, 2000), 30–60; Pernille Hermann, "Literacy," in *The Routledge Research Companion to the Medieval Icelandic Sagas*, ed. Ármann Jakobsson and Sverrir Jakobsson (Routledge, 2017), 34–47.

 | HTTPS://DOI.ORG/10.1163/9789004765528-006

appear, are represented, and are interpreted in the Scandinavian tradition.[6] The sources for studying ritual practices in medieval Scandinavia are therefore primarily textual, with material evidence playing a lesser role. While all of these sources can provide valuable insights and may preserve traces of pre-Christian traditions, however, their reliability needs to be considered carefully within context.[7]

Wthin Old Norse mythological tradition, graphophagy seems to have held a significant place in Germanic and Nordic cultural imaginaries. A particularly instructive example is found in *Sigrdrífumál* ("The Lay of Sigrdrífa"), preserved in the *Poetic Edda*, a corpus of Old Norse poems transmitted in the Icelandic manuscript known as *Codex Regius* (*c.*1270). The poem is primarily didactic in character, much of its content consisting of Sigrdrífa imparting wisdom to the hero Sigurðr. Although extant only in its thirteenth-century written form, *Sigrdrífumál* is generally understood to have circulated orally for several centuries, likely undergoing transmission and adaptation throughout the Viking Age (*c.*800–1050) before its eventual codification.

After slaying the dragon Fáfnir and claiming his immense hoard of gold, Sigurðr sets out on a journey that will shape his fate. Guided by his horse Grani, he rides across the wilderness until he reaches Hindarfjall, a mountain shrouded in myth. There, on its summit, he discovers a valkyrie lying motionless in full armour, surrounded by a wall of fire. When Sigurðr removes the warrior's helmet, he realises that the figure before him is the strikingly beautiful Sigrdrífa, often identified with Brynhildr. She had once defied Óðinn by granting victory to the wrong warrior and, as punishment, had been cast into an enchanted sleep. She was destined to remain thus until awakened by a hero brave enough to ride through the encircling flames.

Upon being awakened, Sigrdrífa expresses her gratitude to Sigurðr by imparting to him an extensive body of knowledge, including the secrets of runes, potent spells, and moral guidance.[8] These teachings are meant to prepare him for his future heroic endeavours and to secure his success. Before introducing him to runic lore, she offers him a *minnisveig* ("memory-drink") to strengthen his recollection.[9] She then provides a drink made from honey

---

6 Judith Jesch, "Runes and Verse: The Medialities of Early Scandinavian Poetry," *European Journal of Scandinavian Studies* 47, no. 1 (2017): 181–202.

7 Stephen A. Mitchell, "Scandinavia," in *The Routledge History of Medieval Magic*, 136–49.

8 Gad Rausing, "On the origin of the runes," *Fornvännen* 87 (1992): 200–205; François-Xavier Dillmann, "Runenmeister," *Reallexikon der Germanischen Altertumskunde*, vol. 25 (de Gruyter, 2003), 537–46.

9 *Sigrdrífumál*, in *Eddukvæði*, ed. Jónas Kristjánsson and Vésteinn Ólason, 2 vols. (Hið íslenzka bókmenntafélag, 2014), II, 313–21, st. 2.

and fruit (*bjór*), infused with special songs (*ljóða*), healing staves (*líknstafa*), charms (*galdra*), and pleasure-runes (*gamanrúna*).[10]

In stanzas 13–14, Sigrdrífa recounts the origins of powerful runes, describing how Hroptr (Óðinn) crafted them from a liquid that dripped from Heiðdraupnir's skull and Hoddrofnir's horn. These runes were then shaved from the carved surfaces and mixed with *helga mjǫð* ("holy mead")[11] before being distributed among gods, elves, and humans:

> All were shaved off, those which were carved on,
> and stirred into the sacred mead
> and sent on wandering ways;
> they are among the Æsir, they are among the elves,
> some are with the wise Vanir,
> some with humankind.[12]

The surfaces upon which runes were inscribed varied widely and included sword hilts, horns, the palms and backs of hands, nails, horse hooves, ships, tree bark, shields, sleighs, animal claws, and bird beaks, among others. Often, the choice of surface and the intended effect appear to have followed the logic of sympathy – for instance, runes carved onto a sword to secure victory in battle.[13]

Particularly noteworthy are passages in *Grágás* – the corpus of laws of the Icelandic Free State laws in force until the 1260s – which refer to individuals who performed "things with stones" or endowed them with specific powers, possibly for the benefit of people or livestock. Such references may point to the use of stones inscribed with runes or other symbols, although the evidence

---

10 Ibid., st. 5. See also Mindy MacLeod and Bernard Mees, *Runic Amulets and Magic Objects* (The Boydell Press, 2006), 239.

11 On this mead and the related motif, see John Stephens, "The Mead of Poetry: Myth and Metaphor," *Neophilologus* 56, no. 3 (1972): 259–68.

12 *Sigrdrífumál*, st. 18: "Allar váru af skafnar, / þær er váru á ristnar, ok hverfðar við inn helga mjöð / ok sendar á víða vega; / þær ro með ásum, / þær ro með alfum, / sumar með vísum vönum / sumar hafa mennskir menn." Trans.: "The Lay of Sigrdrifa," in *The Poetic Edda*, trans. Carolyne Larrington (Oxford University Press, 2014), 162–8. See also Kate Heslop, "Hearing Voices: Uncanny Moments in the *Íslendingasögur*," *Gripla* XIX (2008): 93–122, at 114; Ead., "Talking Heads: The Mediality of Mímir," in *RE:writing. Medial Perspectives on Textual Culture in the Icelandic Middle Ages*, ed. Kate Heslop and Jürg Glauser (Chronos, 2018), 63–84, at 68–9.

13 Katja Schulz, "Inscriptions in Old Norse Literature," in *Writing Beyond Pen and Parchment. Inscribed Objects in Medieval European Literature*, ed. Ricarda Wagner, Christine Neufeld, and Ludger Lieb (de Gruyter, 2019), 41–62, at 52.

remains indirect.[14] More broadly, what legal sources designate as "magic" or "sorcery" (*fjǫlkynngi*, *gørningar*, and *galdr*)[15] was closely associated with the utterance of specific formulaic words over oneself or an object, and with the worship of heathen entities. Engagement in such practices could incur penalties ranging from lesser outlawry – a three-year period of exile – when no harm was deemed to have resulted, to full outlawry in cases involving injury or danger. The latter entailed permanent exile, confiscation of property, and the legal permissibility of killing the offender without legal repercussions.[16]

In *Sigrdrífumál*, writing is presented as a material object endowed with intrinsic power and firmly tied to the pre-Christian cultural horizon.[17] This poem, however, is not the only Old Norse text to reflect on the origins and significance of writing. In *Hávamál*, another Eddic poem, Óðinn sacrifices himself by hanging from Yggdrasill for nine nights, pierced by his own spear and deprived of food and drink. Through this ordeal he attains access to the well of wisdom and perceives the runes, an insight acquired after imbibing a draught

14 *Grágás: Islændernes lovbog i fristatens tid, udg. efter det kongelige Bibliotheks Haanskrift*, ed. Vilhjálmur Finsen, 2 vols. (Odense Universitetsforlag, 1974 [1852]), I, 23: "Menn scolo eigi fara meþ steina. eþa magna þa til þess at binda á men eþa a fé manna. Ef meɴ trva a steina til heilindis ser. eþa fé. oc varþar fiorbaugs garþ."

15 *Fjǫlkynngi*, lit. "knowing many things" or "many forms of knowledge," is usually translated as either "sorcery," "magic," or "witchcraft," but more specifically implied learning certain "magical" skills and techniques. *Galdr* is usually translated as "spell," "charm," "magic," "witchcraft," or "sorcery." It implied the use of runes, staves, verbal and written formulae and incantations (including eating/drinking spells). It seems to have been practiced by both men and women. *Gørningar* was a less common term which referred to some kind of man's interference with the forces of nature. On these forms of magic, see: François-Xavier Dillmann, *Les magiciens dans l'Islande ancienne. Études sur la représentation de la magie islandaise et de ses agents dans les sources littéraires norroises* (Kungl. Gustav Adolfs Akademien för svensk folkkultur, 2006); Catharina Raudvere, "*Trolldómr* in Early Medieval Scandinavia," in *Witchcraft and Magic in Europe. Vol. 3. The Middle Ages*, 73–171, at 110–30; Stephen A. Mitchell, *Witchcraft and Magic in the Nordic Middle Ages* (University of Pennsylvania Press, 2011), 30–1 and 164–6; Ármann Jakobsson, *The Troll Inside You. Paranormal Activity in the Medieval North* (Punctum Books, 2017), 66. See also Gaïa Perreaut, "'Þú Eigir Illa Móður:' Of Cunning Kerlings and *fjǫlkynngi* – Disrupting Social Cohesion Through Magic," in *Performing Magic in the Pre-Modern North. Practice and Transgressions*, ed. Jennifer Hemphill, Ségdae Richardson-Read, and Solveig Marie Wang (Palgrave Macmillan, 2024), 215–38.

16 *Grágás*, I, 23: "Ef maþr ferr með galldra eþa gørningar. eþa fiolkýngi. þa ferr hann með fiolkyngi. ef hann queðr þat eþa kennir. eþa lætr queða. at ser eþa at fe sinv. þat varþar honvm fiorbavgs Garþ. [...] Ef maþr ferr með fordæs skap. þat varþar scoggang. þat ero fordæs skapir. ef maþr gérir i orðum sinvm. eþa fiolkyngi sott eþa bana. fe eþa mavnnvm."

17 Judy Quinn, "Verse Form and Voice in Eddic Pomes: The Discourses of *Fáfnismál*," *Arkiv för nordisk filologi* 107 (1992): 100–30, at 114.

of the "precious mead" (*dýra mjaðar*, the mead of poetry). In the same context, he also gains "nine mighty spells" (*fimbulljóð níu*).[18]

In stanza 144, runes – or writing, more broadly – are explicitly linked to rituals and cultic practices aimed at acquiring power.[19] This connection resonates with the idea that literacy often encourages "the growth of magico-religious activity."[20] In societies in which literacy was confined to a restricted elite, writing frequently served as a privileged medium for invoking or channelling supernatural forces.[21] A comparable conception is found in *Vafþrúðnismál*, which describes aspects of Norse cosmogony and portrays runes as a source of privileged knowledge concerning the world and fate, presenting them as divine gifts accessible only to a select few.[22] This notion is further corroborated by inscriptions such as the Noleby runestone (Västergötland, Sweden, dating from late fourth–late sixth century), which states: "Runo fahi raginakundo toj[e'k]a. ... ... Hakoþuz" ("I prepare the suitable divine rune ... for Hakoþuz").[23] Likewise, the Sparlösa runestone (Västergötland, Sweden, ca. ninth century) reads: "Ok rað runaʀ þaʀ rægi[n]kundu <iu> þar, svað Alrikʀ <lubu> faði" ("And interpret the runes of divine origin there ..., that Alríkr <lubu> coloured").[24]

Old Norse representations of graphophagy have often been interpreted as metaphorical expressions of knowledge transmission within a predominantly oral and "liquid" culture, in which learning is conceptualised as a process of assimilation. The Eddic corpus, a collection of Old Norse mythological and heroic poems preserved in medieval Icelandic manuscripts, repeatedly depicts knowledge as a substance that can be imbibed.[25] Mead and other alcoholic

18 *Sigrdrífumál*, st. 138–45.

19 Terje Spurkland, *Norwegian Runes and Runic Inscriptions*, trans. Betsy van der Hoek (The Boydell Press, 2005), 14.

20 Jack Goody, "Introduction," in *Literacy in Traditional Societies*, 1–26, at 16.

21 Ibid., 15–6; Spurkland, *Norwegian Runes*, 11.

22 *Vafþrúðnismál*, in *Eddukvæði*, I, 356–66, st. 42–3.

23 Bernard Mees, "The Noleby inscription and Germanic *rehana," *Arkiv för nordisk filologi* 133 (2018): 5–28. Runic inscription Vg 63 in the 2020 edition of the Scandinavian Runic-text Database, Department of Scandinavian Languages, Uppsala University. http://kulturarvsdata.se/uu/srdb/91ecd18f-de3e-4eb0-972b-d4f90d3c7f8d.

24 Runic inscription Vg 119 in the 2020 edition of the Scandinavian Runic-text Database, Department of Scandinavian Languages, Uppsala University. http://kulturarvsdata.se/uu/srdb/c4182ee4-d4bc-4f1b-ab1c-abb95a16d49f. The reference to "coloured runes" may hint at the practice of reddening them with blood.

25 Judy Quinn, "Liquid Knowledge: Traditional Conceptualisation of Learning in Eddic Poetry," in *Along the Oral-Written Continuum: Types of Texts, Relations and their Implications*, ed. Slavika Rankovič, Leidulf Melve, and Else Mundal (Brepols, 2010), 183–226.

drinks are consistently associated with the acquisition of wisdom,[26] and the *Eddas* imply that such potency could be activated through the ingestion of shavings from surfaces inscribed with sacred formulas.[27]

These representations raise a series of critical questions. Was the transformative power of words a literary construct deliberately projected onto a distant pagan past by later authors? Or do such narratives reflect residual memories of practices that continued to circulate within Christian Scandinavia? If graphophagy was really practised, did it retain its perceived efficacy once embedded in Christian cultural frameworks?

The Italian historian of religion Ernesto de Martino, renowned for his nuanced analysis of magical ritual, argued that societies experiencing crisis tend to turn to priests, magicians, sorcerers, and shamans as intermediaries with the supernatural. He introduced the notion of the "crisis of presence" to describe moments of profound existential and ontological rupture, in which individuals or communities struggle to maintain a sense of coherence and agency in relation to their world.[28] This approach converges with Bronisław Malinowski's functionalist interpretation of magic as a psychological response to anxiety, providing reassurance at both individual and collective levels.[29] Similarly, Marcel Mauss observed that the definition of magic must be grounded in broader social consensus rather than in the beliefs of marginal groups alone.[30] These perspectives prompt a further question: did medieval Germanic and Nordic societies share a sufficiently widespread belief in the transformative power of words to sustain practices such as graphophagy as socially meaningful and efficacious act?

26 Stephens, "The Mead of Poetry"; Stefka G. Eriksen, "'Liquid Knowledge' in Old Norse Literature and Culture," *Viator* 49, no. 2 (2018): 169–97; Andrea Maraschi, "The Impact of Christianization on Identity-Marking Foods in the Medieval North: Between Pagan Survivals, New Dietary Restrictions, and Magic Practice," *Food&History* 17, no. 2 (2020): 153–81, at 169–70.

27 Catharina Raudvere, "The Power of the Spoken Word as Literary Motif and Ritual Practice in Old Norse Literature," *Viking and Medieval Scandinavia* 1 (2005): 179–202, at 191. Old Norse literature features numerous examples of powers that could be absorbed by eating or drinking. For instance, texts like *Vǫlsunga saga*, *Hrólfs saga kraka*, *Ynglinga saga*, *Þiðriks saga*, *Bósa saga*, and *Dínus saga* describe individuals gaining strength or wisdom through consuming enchanted objects or substances. See Andrea Maraschi, "Eaten Hearts and Supernatural Knowledge in *Eiríks saga rauða*," *Scandia: Journal of Medieval Norse Studies* 1 (2018): 25–47.

28 de Martino, *Il mondo magico*; Id., "Crisi della presenza e integrazione religiosa," *Aut-Aut* 31 (1956): 17–38.

29 Bronisław Malinowski, "Magic, Science and Religion," in Id., *Magic, Science and Religion, and Other Essays*, 17–92, at 62.

30 Mauss, *A General Theory of Magic*, trans. Robert Brain (W.W. Norton, 1972[1902]), 18.

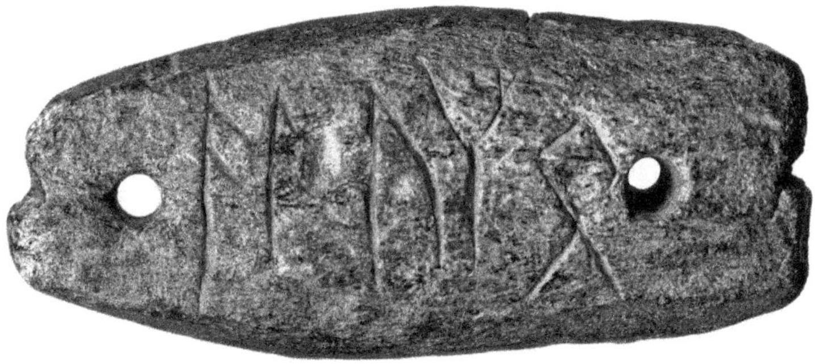

FIGURE 13 Fishing weight inscribed with runes, possibly attributed with special powers. N KJ49, Bergen, University Museum 2929 (side A). Provenance: Førde, Norway. Universitetsmuseet i Bergen

While the sources offer no definitive conclusions, a number of suggestive clues can be traced back to the Roman and Germanic Iron Ages. One such example is a third-to-sixth-century soapstone net-sinker from Western Norway, which seems to imply that runes could activate their efficacy when immersed in water. Measuring 12 cm in length and 5 cm in width, the object is carved with a fish on one side – likely a sympathetic image intended to attract prey (figs. 13–14).[31] On the reverse, a runic inscription reads *aluko*, which may represent either a diminutive form of a female personal name ("Little Alu") or a reference to *alu*, a term often interpreted as bearing magico-religious significance.[32]

Similar talismans have been found outside of Scandinavia as well. Two further examples are described in the mid-tenth-century Arabic handbook of natural magic, the *Ghāyat al-hakīm* (to be discussed in greater detail below).[33] The first talisman was made by drawing a fish's head, body, and tail "in the hour of Venus and in the ascendant of Pisces when Jupiter is in it," assembling the image on a silver rod placed in a lead bowl filled with water, and finally submerging the vessel in a river to attract fish.[34] The second talisman involved drawing a fish "in the hour of the Moon and in the ascendant of the first phase

31 See Sophus Bugge and Magnus Olsen, *Norges Indskrifter med de ældre Runer. Inledning*, 3 vols. (Brøgger, 1891–1924), vol. 1, n. 24, 312–5.

32 Bernard Mees, *The English Language Before England. An Epigraphic Account* (Routledge, 2023), 187–9.

33 *Picatrix, Ghayat al-Hakim, The Goal of the Wise*, I, 39 and 41.

34 Venus and Jupiter were in a peculiar reciprocal connection, for "Venus might respond to what was asked from Jupiter and Jupiter might respond to what was asked from Venus" (ibid., II, 205). Venus, in particular, could grant any wish (ibid., II, 111). Silver, in turn, was associated with the Moon (ibid., I, 123 and II, 9).

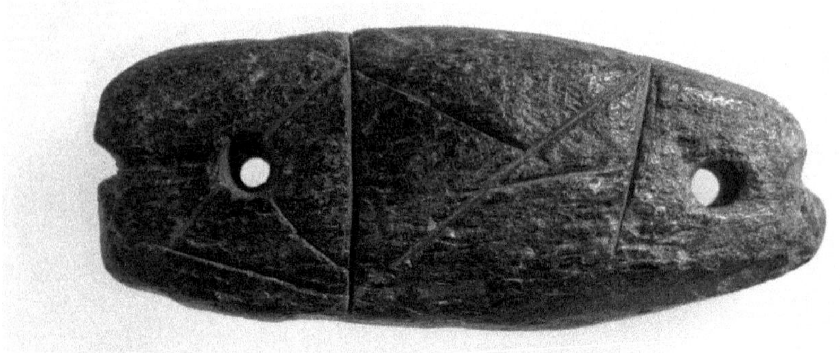

FIGURE 14 Side B of the same. N KJ49, Bergen, University Museum 2929. Universitetsmuseet i Bergen (Photo by Svein Skare)

of Pisces, within which are the Moon and Mercury." In this case, the act of drawing alone, when performed under the appropriate planetary configuration, was sufficient to endow the image with natural power – Pisces being understood to exercise dominion over aquatic creatures.[35]

Another intriguing artifact was discovered at Fløksand, Norway, dating to the fourth century CE (fig. 15).[36] Recovered from a cremation urn in a female grave, the knife bears the runic inscription *lina laukR f*. The term *lina* means "linen" or "flax," while *laukR* refers to "leek" or a related plant, which appears in *Sigrdrífumál* (stanza 8) as an antidote to magical poisons. The *f* rune, corresponding to "wealth" or "cattle" in the Elder Futhark, further strengthens the interpretation of the inscription as possessing an extra-linguistic, potentially apotropaic or efficacious, dimension.[37]

Comparable examples are attested elsewhere in Europe in this case as well. Remedies for insomnia recorded since the second half of the ninth century attest to the practice of inscribing specific words on the handle of a knife – such as *fres*, *refres*, *perfres*, and *serperis*, or variants including *fres refres*, and *profres*, or *reres*, *refers*, *proferes*, and *referes* – which was then dipped and placed on or beneath the head of the patient without their knowledge.[38]

35 Ibid., II, 14.

36 See Bugge and Olsen, *Norges Indskrifter*, vol. 2, n. 51, 648–52; Wolfgang Krause and Herbert Jankuhn, *Die Runeninschriften im älteren Futhark* (Vandenhoeck and Ruprecht, 1966), n. 37.

37 John McKinnell, Rudolf Simek, and Klaus Düwel, *Runes, Magic and Religion. A Sourcebook* (Fassbaender, 2004), 97–8.

38 St. Gallen, Stiftsbibliothek, 751, p. 434: "Ad somnu*m* mirificam rem. Scribe in manico cultelli at ferro incipie*ns* bis: fres refres p*ro*fres serperis, q*uo*d nescienti ad caput ponis et de una tincta fiat"; British Library, Sloane MS 475, fol. 26r: "Ad illu*m* q*ui* n*on* dormit

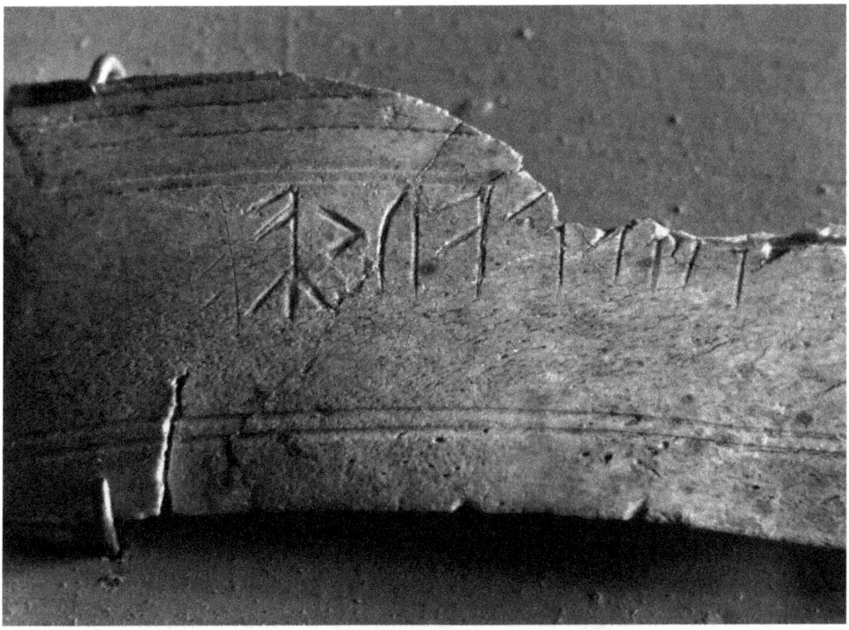

FIGURE 15 Bone tool (knife/scraper) from Fløksand, with Elder Futhark runic inscription "lin(al)aukaz(?)"; burial find, 4th century AD. N KJ37, Bergen, University Museum B1792. Universitetsmuseet i Bergen

The aforementioned Scandinavian inscriptions, along with those found on bracteates, suggest a ritualistic intent, possibly aimed at invoking fertility or health through the instrumentality of the knife.[39] Related examples also appear in the Anglo-Saxon medical tradition.[40] The formula *lina laukar* is relatively widespread in runic carvings and has frequently been associated with

probate res. Scribe in manubrio cultelli a ferro incipiens: reres refers proferes referes, et illi nescienti ad cap*u*t pones de intincta script*um* in abbo manubrio cultelli afferro incipiens"; Bern, Burgerbibliothek, Cod. 803, fol. 1r: "Ad somnum. Scribe in mantico cultelli ferrum incipiens: fres, refres, profres, quod nescienti quod caput pone et de una intinctione fiat."

39 See Raymond I. Page, *Runes and Runic Inscriptions: Collected Essays On Anglo-Saxon and Viking Runes* (The Boydell Press, 1995), 106–8; Tineke Looijenga, *Texts & Contexts of the Oldest Runic Inscriptions* (Brill, 2003), 199. The practice of inscribing letters on knives is found elsewhere in Europe, as in the aforementioned scroll from southern Alsace, Bern, Burgerbibliothek, Cod. 803, fol. 1r: "Ad somnum. Scribe in mantico cultelli ad ferr*um* incipiens. fres. refres. p*ror*fres. q*uo*d nescienti ad caput pone et de una intinctione fiat;" and, similarly on the recto: "Ad p*ro*fluiu*m* mulieris. Scribe tales caracteres et sub pectine pone et si n*on* credis scribe i*n* cultello et iacula porcellu*m* cu*m* eo et sanguis n*on* exit ..."

40 Storms, *Anglo-Saxon Magic*, 237, 249, 257, and 287.

magical efficacy or with specific cultic contexts. Furthermore, linen, leeks, and onions were commonly used in food preparation as preserving agents. Leeks, in particular, were widely employed in medical practice and were often attributed fertility-related properties, partly owing to their phallic form.

What matters for graphophagy is the trajectory: runic inscriptions on portable objects that touch skin, clothing, or (in the knife's case) food being prepared. The boundary between wearing and ingesting runic power seems to have been permeable: an inscribed knife used to cut food transfers runic power into what is eaten and – through sympathetic logic – back into the environment, possibly attracting or ensuring future abundance of the same type of food. It represents a case of power transfer through material contiguity rather than direct consumption, as seen in other cases mentioned above.

Archaeological evidence from medieval Scandinavia indicates that runes believed to possess healing powers were carved onto wooden sticks, among other objects. Comparable practices are described in medieval Icelandic sagas, although these accounts may serve specific narratological purposes and must be approached with due caution. While some scholars argue that such accounts can only inform us of their authors' contemporary views of runic power, others deem them valuable – though not entirely reliable – sources.[41] For instance, *Egils saga Skalla-Grímssonar*, likely composed between 1230 and 1240, portrays a protagonist deeply associated with runic knowledge.[42] Egill, both farmer and skald, embodies the saga's unique emphasis on runes and their practical application. Unlike many other *Íslendingasögur*, *Egils saga* underscores the materiality of runes and the necessity of precise and informed usage.

A pivotal episode regarding runes unfolds at a farm on Atley Island, managed by a man named Bárðr. The estate belonged to the Norwegian king Eiríkr blóðøx (Bloodaxe) and his queen, Gunnhildr. At first, Egill's presence goes unnoticed, and Bárðr offers him bread, butter, and bowls of curds and whey.

41 Judith Jesch and Christina Lee, "Healing runes," in *Viking Encounters*, ed. Anne Pedersen and Søren Sindbæk (Aarhus University Press, 2020), 386–98. On "magic" in the sagas, see: Stephen A. Mitchell, "Magic as Acquired Art and the Ethnographic Value of the Sagas," in *Old Norse Myths, Literature and Society*, ed. Margaret Clunies Ross (University Press of Southern Denmark, 2003), 132–52; Mitchell, *Witchcraft and Magic*, 74–116.

42 On this saga, see: Torfi H. Tulinius, *The Matter of the North. The Rise of Literary Fiction in Thirteenth-Century Iceland*, trans. Randi C. Eldevik (Odense University Press, 2002), 234–89; Id., "Egils saga and the novel," in *Snorri Sturluson and the Roots of Nordic Literature: Papers of the International Conference held at "St. Kliment Ohridski" University of Sofia (October 14–16, 2002)* (University of Sofia, 2002), 117–28; Id., "The Construction of Egil's Saga," in *Egil, the Viking Poet: New Approaches to 'Egils saga'*, ed. Laurence de Looze, Jón Karl Helgason, Russell Poole, and Torfi H. Tulinius (University of Toronto Press, 2015), 23–39.

Meanwhile, King Eiríkr is hosting a feast elsewhere, with abundant strong ale, and has Egill summoned to his hall. During the feast, Egill – ever wary due to his turbulent past – suspects that the ale offered to him may be poisoned, a fear not unfounded given the hostility between himself and Bárðr. Furthermore, the Norwegian royal family was embroiled in conflict with Egill's kin, and Gunnhildr regarded Egill as a dangerous and uncontrollable adversary of her husband. For this reason, she and Bárðr conspire to poison his drink. To test its safety, Egill draws upon his runic expertise: he carves runes into his drinking horn, smears them with his own blood, and recites a skaldic verse invoking their power to reveal the true nature of the ale. Upon completing the incantation, the horn shatters, thereby confirming that the drink had indeed been poisoned:[43]

> Egill took out his knife and stabbed the palm of his hand with it, then took the drinking-horn, carved runes on it and smeared them with blood. He spoke a verse:
>
> I carve runes on this horn,
> redden words with my blood,
> I choose words for the trees
> of the wild beast's ear-roots;
> drink as we wish this mead
> brought by merry serving maids,
> let us find out how we fare
> from the ale that Bárðr blessed.
>
> The horn shattered and the drink spilled onto the straw.[44]

This act not only saves Egill from harm but also consolidates his reputation as a master of runic powers and *seiðr* – a term denoting an archaic divinatory and ritual art originally associated with the goddess Freyja and later linked to

43 On the hagiographic parallel in Gregory the Great's *Dialogi*, see Siân Grønlie, "Saint's Life and Saga Narrative," *Saga-Book* XXXVI (2012): 5–26.

44 *Egils saga*, ed. Bjarni Einarsson (Viking Society for Northern Research, 2003), 59: "Egill brá þá knífi sínum ok stakk í lófa sér; hann tók við horninu ok reist á rúnar ok reið á blóðinu. Hann kvað: Rístum rún á horni, / rjóðum spjǫll í dreyra, / þau velk orð til eyrna / óðs dýrs viðar róta; / drekkum veig sem viljum, / vel glýjaðra þýja; / vita, hvé oss of eiri / ǫl þat er Bárðr of signdi. / Hornit sprakk í sundr, en drykkrinn fór niðr í hálm." Trans.: Bernard Scudder, *Egils Saga*, in *The Complete Sagas of the Icelanders, Including 49 Tales*, ed. Viðar Hreinsson, 5 vols. (Leifur Eiríksson, 1997), I, 33–177, at 82.

practices perceived as dangerous or morally suspect.[45] Within the narrative economy of the saga, the episode fulfils several functions: it highlights Egill's intellectual acuity, underscores the atmosphere of mistrust and enduring conflict among the characters, and illustrates the cultural centrality of runes within Old Norse mythological and literary discourse. This interplay between feud, runic power, and poetic performance is, in this respect, fundamental to *Egils saga*.

Egill's mastery of runes is further emphasised on two more occasions. The first occurs when he erects a *níðstǫng* ("insult pole") against king Eiríkr, combining a carved inscription with the severed head of a horse – an act that the saga connects with Eiríkr's subsequent exile to York.[46] The second episode unfolds when Egill encounters runes carved onto a whalebone by an inexperienced farmer. Intended as a love charm, the inscription instead causes the woman concerned to fall ill.[47] Recognising both the danger and the misuse of runic knowledge, Egill erases the runes and burns the material, thereby underscoring the importance of expertise in rune carving – a competence for which

---

45 William Sayers, "Poetry and Social Agency in *Egils saga Skalla-Grímssonar*," *Scripta Islandica* 45 (1995): 29–62; Neil Price, *The Viking Way: Religion and War in Late Iron Age Scandinavia* (Uppsala universitet, Department of Archaeology and Ancient History, 2002). On the connections between Egill's runes and typical Old Norse runic inscriptions, see Margaret Clunies Ross, "Self-Description in Egil's Poetry," in *Egil, the Viking Poet*, 75–91, esp. 84–5; Laurence De Looze, "Poet, Poem and Poetic Process in Egils Saga *Skalla-Grímssonar*," *Arkiv för nordisk filologi* 104 (1989): 123–42. On *seiðr*, Clive Tolley, *Shamanism in Norse Myth and Magic*. 2 vols. (Academia Scientiarum Fennica, 2009), 423; Eldar Heide, "Spinning *seiðr*," in *Old Norse religion in long-term perspectives. Origins, changes, and interactions*, ed. Anders Andrén, Kristina Jennbert, and Catharina Raudvere (Nordic Academic Press, 2006), 164–70; François-Xavier Dillmann, "Seiður og shamanismi í Íslendingasögum," *Skáldskaparmál* 2 (1993): 20–33; Nicolas Meylan, *Magic and Kingship in Medieval Iceland. The Construction of a Discourse of Political Resistance* (Brepols, 2014), 39.

46 *Egils saga*, 98: "Hann tók í hǫnd sér heslistǫng ok gekk á bergsnǫs nǫkkura þá er vissi til lands inn; þá tók hann hrosshǫfuð ok setti upp á stǫngina. Síðan veitti hann formála ok mælti svá: 'Hér set ek upp níðstǫng ok sný ek þessu níði á hǫnd Eiríki konungi ok Gunnhildi dróttningu' – hann sneri hrosshǫfðinu inn á land, – 'sný ek þessu níði á landvættir þær er land þetta byggja svá at allar fari þær villar vega, engi hendi né hitti sitt inni fyrr en þær reka Eirík konung ok Gunnhildi ór landi.' Síðan skýtr hann stǫnginni niðr í bjargrifu ok lét þar standa. Hann sneri ok hǫfðinu inn á land, en hann reist rúnar á stǫnginni ok segja þær formála þenna allan."

47 *Egils saga*, 136–7: "Skalat maðr rúnar rísta / nema ráða vel kunni. / Þat verðr mǫrgum manni / er um myrkvan staf villisk. / Sá ek á telgðu tálkni / tíu launstafi ristna. / Þat hefir lauka lindi / langs oftrega fengit"; and 142: "þá þóttisk <hann> rísta henni manrúnar, en hann kunni þat eigi ok hafði hann þat ristit henni er hon fekk meinsemi af."

he is renowned. The saga thus presents runic practice as a specialised craft, fraught with risk and unsuitable for the untrained.

The perceived potency of runes is further exemplified in *Skírnismál*, where Skírnir, a servant of Freyr, seeks to win the giantess Gerðr for his master. When persuasion fails, he switches to threats, invoking runic magic and warning that he will carve runes onto a horn as part of a curse.[48] The episode implies that runic power inheres in the inscriptions themselves, independent of the carver's intention or depth of understanding.[49] Such assumptions find a revealing counterpart in *Hávamál* stanza 144, in which Óðinn asks: "Veiztu hvé rísta skal? Veiztu hvé ráða skal?" ("Do you know how to carve? Do you know how to interpret?"),[50] thus stressing the necessity of technical skill and interpretative competence. It has been argued that Skírnir's curse may reflect actual practices, as archaeological evidence seems to suggest.[51]

Other Old Norse sources imply that words – both spoken and written – possessed a tangible capacity to reshape reality. Icelandic authors, including Snorri Sturluson, exploit this conceptual framework in works such as *Ynglinga saga* and the *Prose Edda*.[52] In *Ynglinga saga*, Snorri describes how Óðinn could extinguish fires, still the sea, and govern the winds through *ljóð* (chants) known as *galdrar*, leading to the Æsir being called *galdrasmíðir* ("spell-smiths") and *ljóðasmíðir* ("song-smiths").[53]

While *skáldskapr* (poetry) was socially sanctioned, *seiðr* was formally condemned; nonetheless, both were understood to partake of supernatural efficacy. In *Egils saga*, Egill's seating in the second high-seat at the royal court reflects the considerable esteem accorded to Icelandic poets. Over time, however, the prestige of skaldic poetry waned. During the reign of King Magnús

48 *Skírnismál*, in *Eddukvæði*, I, 380–88, st. 36.

49 Cardona, *Antropologia della scrittura*.

50 *Hávamál*, in *Eddukvæði*, II, 322–55, st. 144.

51 Runic inscription N B257 in the 2020 edition of the Scandinavian Runic-text Database, Department of Scandinavian Languages, Uppsala University. http://kulturarvsdata.se/uu/srdb/c0162b72-0be1-4841-be92-f2a618300db9. See Stephen A. Mitchell, "*Skírnismál* and Nordic Charm Magic," in *Reflections on Old Norse Myths*, ed. Pernille Hermann, Jens Peter Schjødt, and Rasmus Tranum Kristensen (Brepols, 2007), 75–94, esp. 85–6; Daniel Sävborg, "Painful Love and Desire in Skírnismál: Origins and Contexts," in *The Wild Hunt for Numinous Knowledge: Perspectives on and from the Study of Pre-Christian Nordic Religion in Honour of Jens Peter Schjødt*, ed. Karen Bek-Pedersen, Sophie Bønding, Luke John Murphy, Simon Nygaard, and Morten Warmind, *Religionsvidenskabeligt Tidsskrift* 74 (2022): 490–512.

52 Meylan, "The Magical Power."

53 Snorri Sturluson, *Ynglinga saga*, in *Heimskringla* I, ed. Bjarni Aðalbjarnarson, Íslenzk fornrít XXVI (Hið íslenska bókmenntafélag, 1941), 9–83.

Erlingsson (1161–84), the Norwegian monarchy increasingly grounded its legitimacy in written texts rather than oral tradition, further weakening the social function of skalds.[54] This process continued under King Hákon Hákonarson (1217–63), whose patronage of translated French and English romances further marginalised traditional skaldic poetry.[55] This cultural shift – experienced firsthand by Snorri Sturluson – may have prompted saga authors to reinforce the conceptual links between poetry, *seiðr*, *fjǫlkynngi*, and *galdr*. By doing so, these texts sought not merely to preserve memory but to reaffirm the historical prestige of poets and the enduring, transformative potency attributed to language itself.

Notably, the medieval Icelandic law code *Grágás* addresses both love and blame poetry, stipulating that the former could exert influence over a woman's will, while the latter could harm a man's honour – offences punishable by fines and, in more serious cases, by outlawry.[56] The legal texts, however, draw no explicit connection between poetry and magic. Within this juridical framework, the effects of verse depended on its content rather than on the identity or intent of its composer. Prose, notably, was not regarded as potentially dangerous. By the time *Egils saga* was composed, the perceived potency of words – whether operating in legal, social, or magical domains – thus remained a matter of active cultural concern.

References to carved horns imbued with supernatural properties also occur in *Guðrúnarkviða II* and *Vǫlsunga saga*, where Guðrún is given an *uminnisveig* ("drink of oblivion").[57] After consuming this potion, she forgets her grief and consents to marry King Atli. The horn is described as being engraved with "all manner of letters" (*stafir*), which are stained with blood, while the ale it contains is mixed with a range of ingredients, including herbs, burnt acorns, soot, sacrificial entrails, and boiled pig's liver. Saxo Grammaticus recounts a similar episode in which a giantess inscribes *carmina* (runic spells) onto a piece of wood and places it beneath a dead man's tongue, thereby enabling him to

54 Sverre Bagge, *From Gang Leader to the Lord's Anointed. Kingship in Sverris saga and Hákonar saga Hákonarsonar* (Syddansk universitetsforlag, 1996).

55 Kevin Wanner, *Snorri Sturluson and the Edda. The Conversion of Cultural Capital in Medieval Scandinavia* (University of Toronto Press, 2008), 73ff.

56 *Grágás*, I, 183–4. See also Anne Holtsmark, "Kjærlighetsdiktning," in *Kulturhistorisk leksikon for nordisk middelalder*, ed. Johannes Brøndsted et al., 22 vols. (Rosenkilde og Bagger, 1956–78), VIII, 438–43.

57 *Guðrúnarkviða II*, in *Eddukvæði*, II, 352–61, st. 22; *Völsunga saga*, in *Fornaldar sögur Norðurlanda*, 4 vols., ed. Guðni Jónsson (Íslendingasagnaútgáfan, 1954), I, 107–218, ch. 32. On the existence and use of such horns, see Anne Hofmann, "Drinking Horns in Old Norse Culture: A Tradition Under Examination," *Analecta Archaeologica Ressoviensia* 10 (2015): 214–70.

speak.[58] This narrative closely parallels *Hávamál*, where Óðinn describes a runic spell capable of reanimating the dead and compelling them to speak.[59]

One of the principal challenges in studying graphophagy in the Old Norse context lies in the lack of continuous and chronologically coherent sources documenting its practice across time. It may be therefore be tempting to dismiss graphophagy as a purely literary motif devised by Christian Icelandic authors to construct a symbolic bridge to a pagan past, or to interpret it exclusively as a metaphor for the transmission of knowledge, as Judy Quinn has suggested with regard to the Eddic poems.[60] Nevertheless, as this book seeks to demonstrate, a range of textual, legal, and material sources indicates that graphophagy was not merely a narrative conceit but formed part of a broader repertoire of practices attested in early and high medieval Europe.

As has been observed in other regions, later sources are valuable for establishing a wider perspective and for tracing the continuity of such practices. In late medieval Scandinavia, leechbooks and collections of charms preserve remedies that are clearly rooted in graphophagy.[61] It is, of course, possible that this tradition of graphophagic practices in late medieval Scandinavian medical and magical texts was almost entirely influenced by their respective sources, which had long been circulating in the West. Nevertheless, the Scandinavian cultural background may have been particularly receptive to such practices, inasmuch as the power of writing and references to graphophagy were notions that – through the mythological and poetic heritage and their later literary iterations – were themselves very ancient and well established. Particularly significant manuscripts include AM 187 8 ° (a Danish medical treatise, fourteenth–fifteenth century), Royal Irish Academy 23 D 43 (an Icelandic medical miscellany, late fifteenth century), AM 434a 12mo (an Icelandic charms collection, fifteenth century), and Linköping Stifts Bibliotek M5 (a Swedish medical text, *c.*1500). Taken together, these sources attest to the enduring reliance on graphophagic practices within medico-religious contexts.

For instance, a remedy *ad solucionem uentris* ("to loosen the bowels") in AM 187 8 ° prescribes writing the formula *currens discurrit cursur, conseruat*

58 Saxo Grammaticus, *Gesta Danorum. Danmarkshistorien*, ed. Karsten Friis-Jensen, trans. Peter Zeeberg, 2 vols. (Danske Sprog- og Litteraturselskab & Gads Forlag, 2005), I, 1.6.3, 46: "Ubi magice speculationis officio superum mentem rimari cupiens, diris admodum carminibus ligno insculptis iisdemque linguae defuncti per Hadingum suppositis, hac voce eum horrendum auribus carmen edere coegit …".

59 *Hávamál*, in *Eddukvæði*, II, 322–55, st. 157.

60 The use of runes is clearly associated with the pre-Christian past in *Grettis saga*, for instance (ch 79). Schulz, "Inscriptions," 51.

61 Maraschi, "Sympathetic Graphophagy."

utrumque famulus dei on an apple or a loaf of bread and then feeding it to the patient.[62] The phrase *currens discurrit cursur* functions as a form of sympathetic writing, repeatedly urging the intestines to release their contents, while *famulus dei* ("servant of God," commonly used to address saints) establishes an explicit link with divine authority. This manuscript reflects the influence of the so-called "Danish Salernitan" Henrik Harpestræng (d. 1244), the most prominent figure in medieval Danish medicine.[63] Although Harpestræng's herbal treatises draw heavily on the traditions of the *Schola Medica Salernitana* and humoral theory, they include a few remedies involving prayers charms, in keeping with broader European medical practice. A similar procedure appears in a remedy *vid nef dreyra* ("for nosebleed") in Royal Irish Academy 23 D 43, an encyclopaedic compilation representing the largest extant medical manuscript in Norse.[64] Here, the words *consummatum est*, drawn from John 19:30, are to be written on the patient's forehead using the patient's own blood.[65] The blood is then washed off with water, collected in a cup, and given to the patient to drink while the verse is recited aloud.[66]

Commonly used surfaces include apples, bread (both loaves and consecrated wafers), leeks or onions, cheese, fish, and earth – materials chosen for their ready availability and the ease with which they could be inscribed, ensuring the legibility of the signs. Alternatively, patients were instructed to ingest the

62 Viggo Såby, ed., *Det arnamagnæanske handskrift nr. 187 i ocktav, indeholdende en dansk lægebog* (Thieles Bogtrykkeri, 1883), 71: "Ite*m* Ad solucione*m* uentris. Scribe i*n* pomo aut i*n* pane *et* da *co*medere. Om thu wilt hauæ mikæl løfn i thin quid, scrijf th*æt*tæ abrøth æller a æplæ, oc æt th*æt*: Currens discurrit cursur, *con*seruat utru*m*q*ue* famulus dei."

63 J.W.S. Johnsson, "Henrik Harpestraeng. A Danish Salernitan," *Isis* 4, no. 1 (1921): 13–16. On the manuscript, see John Kousgård Sørensen, "Lægebøger," *Kulturhistorisk leksikon for nordisk middelalder* 2:2 (1982): 76–79, at 77; Thelma Jexlev, *Lokalarkiver til 1559: Gejstlige arkiver*, Bd. I: *Ærkestiftet og Roskilde stift*, Bd. 2: *Odense stift, jyske stifter og Slesvig stift. Rigsarkivet* (Rigsarkivet, 1973–1977), I, 288.

64 Henning Larsen, ed., *An Old Icelandic Medical Miscellany. MS Royal Irish Academy 23 D 43* (Dybwad, 1931), 1–2.

65 "Cum ergo accepisset Iesus acetum dixit consummatum est, et inclinato capite tradidit spiritum" ("When he had received the drink, Jesus said, 'It is finished.' With that, he bowed his head and gave up his spirit").

66 Ibid., 50: "Tak blod*it ok* rita j en*ne* h*o*nu*m* ok þvo sid*an* of*an* j vatn *ok* gef h*o*nu*m* at d*r*ecka *ok* les sid*an* *con*sumatu*m* *est*." Comparable principles recur in the early modern Icelandic grimoire *Galdrabók* (MS ATA, Ämbetsarkiv 2, Vitterhetsakademiens handskriftsamling, serie F 16 v. 26). The text contains instructions for inscribing *galdrastafir* onto foodstuffs or dissolving them into drinks. *En isländsk svartkonstbok från 1500-talet* (*Galdrabók*), ed. Natan Lindqvist (Appelbergs boktryckeri aktiebolag, 1921), 50. See Andrea Maraschi, "Nature, Supernature and the Human Body. Medicinal Remedies and Charms in Late Medieval Scandinavia," in *(Extra)Ordinary Bodies: Othered, Violated, and Devoured*, ed. Andrea Maraschi and Angelica A. Montanari (Bookstones, 2023), 70–80.

ink used to write biblical verses or other sacred formulas. Several of the other substances employed were everyday staples in Scandinavian households. This suggests that graphophagic practices did not require exotic ingredients and that the boundary between learned and popular practice was likely porous. At the same time, such evidence reinforces the plausibility of *Egils saga* in attributing power to both inscribed words and to their users – regardless of the identity of the inscriber – and highlights the potentially hazardous nature of these practices within their cultural context.

Neil Price has observed that "the understanding of runes as magical signs ultimately rests almost entirely on the written sources."[67] While such sources should not be underestimated, he notes that they mainly demonstrate the centrality of runes within the internal logic of Viking-Age ritual, rather than providing unequivocal evidence for their specific operative functions. He therefore cautions against relying on literary sources alone to draw definitive conclusions about the magical uses of runes in contrast to their more prosaic applications. This methodological caution is well founded. At the same time, the numerous traces of graphophagic practices across medieval Europe must be taken into account. Although the archaeological record does not offer definitive proof that runes were employed exactly as described in *Sigrdrífumál* and related texts, the medieval North constituted a cultural milieu in which references to such practices were far from exceptional. Whether Old Norse descriptions of these practices can be considered reliable remains a key question. Despite their appeal, such sources often reflect their authors' (re)constructions of the past rather than faithful representations of earlier practices. Yet, as Stephen Mitchell has argued, many of the Christian authors who committed the Eddic corpus and the sagas to writing were themselves culturally embedded in Northern European cultures and "possessed more emic views than we sometimes credit them with."[68]

Fictional narratives and documentary evidence cannot, of course, be treated as epistemologically equivalent, as narrative sources offer mediated representations of the past. Nevertheless, in the particular case of graphophagy, literary and historical sources partially overlap, suggesting the persistence and continued intelligibility of a pre-Christian conceptual framework.[69]

67 Neil Price, *The Viking Way. Magic and Mind in Late Iron Age Scandinavia* (Oxbow, 2019), 62.

68 Stephen A. Mitchell, "Magic and Religion," in *The Pre-Christian Religions of the North. History and Structures, Volume I: Basic Premises and Consideration of Sources*, ed. Jens Peter Schjødt, John Lindow, and Anders Andrén (Brepols, 2020), 643–70, at 646.

69 On *Egils saga* in particular, see Torfi H. Tulinius, *The Enigma of Egill. The Saga, the Viking poet, and Snorri Sturluson*, trans. Victoria Cribb (Cornell University Library, 2014), 138.

Within this framework, spoken and written words – when carved, scraped, and ingested – were seemingly believed to possess the capacity to effect tangible change in reality, a notion that continued to resonate in legal discourse well into the Christian period.

The Nordic world was embedded in extensive networks of contact linking Scandinavia to western Europe and the eastern Mediterranean, making the transmission of beliefs and practices attested from Ireland to the Mediterranean basin entirely plausible[70] – particularly where such practices were grounded in broadly shared notions of cosmic sympathy. In light of the agents involved and the narrative contexts in which graphophagy appears in Old Norse sources, the practice was perceived as having remote, mythic origins. Scandinavian leechbooks and collections of charms further indicate that graphophagy persisted into the late medieval and early modern periods, paralleling its continued circulation elsewhere in Europe. Collectively, the sources point to the prestige of a practice that had circulated among diverse populations over many centuries, representing a marginal yet resilient human strategy for confronting uncertainty, illness, and misfortune.

70 Jesch and Lee, "Healing runes." See also Roberto Pagani, "The Mediterranean Origin of the *Galdrastafir*. Tracing the Transmission of the Learned European Magical Tradition into Icelandic Popular Lore," *Gripla* 36 (2025): 241–69, which focuses on the Mediterranean origins of Icelandic *galdrastafir*.

CHAPTER 5

Mediterranean Paths

During the twelfth century, the city of Salerno stood at the centre of a vibrant intellectual and medical milieu. As a major port, it was home to Christian, Jewish, and Muslim communities, and its close political and commercial ties with Sicily facilitated the transmission of medical texts and practices across linguistic and cultural boundaries.[1] It was in this period that Greek medical writings – long preserved, studied, and expanded within the Arabic-speaking world – began to circulate more widely in western Europe through Latin translation.

The *Schola Medica Salernitana* had by then earned a reputation as one of the foremost centres for medical learning and practice in the Latin West. It was within this context that the influential collection of medical writings conventionally known as *Trotula* was compiled.[2] Consisting of three treatises – *Liber de sinthomatibus mulierum, De curis mulierum*, and *De ornatu mulierum* – the *Trotula* tradition was long attributed to a female practitioner named Trota (or Trocta) and focuses primarily on women's health, reproduction, and bodily care.[3] These texts draw on classical medical authorities as mediated through Arabic translations and commentaries, while simultaneously integrating local therapeutic practices current in southern Italy.[4]

Within this learned yet eclectic medical framework, sympathetic remedies, amulets, and verbal formulae continued to occupy a legitimate place,

1 David Waines, "Dietetics in Medieval Islamic Culture," *Medical History* 43 (1999): 228–40.

2 Monica H. Green, ed., *The* Trotula: *An English Translation of the Medieval Compendium of Women's Medicine* (University of Pennsylvania Press, 2002). By then, Salerno had been an important – though informal – centre for the study of medicine for a few centuries, as the early tenth-century *Regimen Sanitatis Salernitanum* suggests; possibly, the most ancient school of medical knowledge of medieval Europe. See: *La Scuola Medica Salernitana. Gli autori e i testi*, ed. Danielle Jacquart and Agostino Paravicini Bagliani (SISMEL – Edizioni del Galluzzo, 2007); Giovanni Vitolo, "La Scuola medica salernitana come metafora della storia del Mezzogiorno," *Studi Storici* 45, no. 3 (2004): 633–50; Erminio Morenghi, "Trotula de' Ruggiero e la Scuola medica salernitana. Una pioniera della medicina per le donne fatta da una donna," *Italies* 27 (2023): 93–106; *Medieval Medicine. A Reader*, 129. On the genre of the *regimina mensium*, see Francesca Pucci Donati, *Dieta, salute, calendari: dal regime stagionale antico ai* regimina mensium *medievali: origine di un genere nella letteratura medica occidentale* (CISAM, 2007).

3 On the texts' authorship and their cultural context, see Green, ed., *The* Trotula, 1–67.

4 Ibid., 2.

 | HTTPS://DOI.ORG/10.1163/9789004765528-007

especially in the treatment of gynaecological conditions. Whether as a result of this cultural synthesis or as a reflection of long-standing therapeutic habits, such practices persisted alongside humoral explanations and pharmacological interventions. Thus, in the anonymous *Liber de sinthomatibus mulierum* ("Book on the conditions of women"), the author records a remedy intended to assist a woman in labour, which reads as follows:

> Vel scribantur hec nomina in caseo uel butyro: + sa. e. op. ab. z. po. c. zy. e. pe. pa. pu. c. ac. sator arepo tenet os pera rotas, et dentur ad manducandum.[5]

> Or let these names be written on cheese or butter + sa. e. op. ab. z. po. c. zy. e pe. pa. pu. c. ac. sator arepo tenet os pera rotas, and let them be given to eat.

In the event of a delayed pregnancy or if the foetus were stillborn in the womb, then another formula should instead be drunk:

> Quod si adhuc tardet partus uel si fetus mortuus est in ea et non liberatur, bibat a. ii. i. c. r. z. py. di. lac alterius mulieris et statim liberabitur.[6]

> But if birth is up to now still delayed or if the foetus is dead inside her and she is not delivered of it, let her drink a. ii. i. c. r. z. py. di., the milk of another woman and immediately she will be delivered.

These prescriptions are rare but significant examples of graphophagy within the Salernitan tradition and present a number of interpretative challenges. First, the ultimate sources of these remedies remain unknown.[7] The earlier formula, in particular, contains a corrupted version of the well-known *sator-arepo* palindrome (*os pera*). As Monica Green has shown, this version appears only in the so-called proto-ensemble of the *Trotula*, compiled in the late twelfth century, where it replaced an earlier Christian charm. Although the palindromic structure is compromised due to a typo in the text, the formula may have been retained precisely because its efficacy was not thought to depend on semantic intelligibility. Rather, its power resided in its perceived antiquity and in its extra-linguistic qualities.

5 Ibid., 100.
6 Ibid., 102.
7 Monica H. Green, "The Development of the Trotula," *Revue d'Histoire des Textes* 26 (1996): 119–203. Reprinted in: Monica H. Green, *Women's Healthcare in the Medieval West* (Routledge, 2000), 119–203, here 188.

The *sator-arepo* palindrome is attested in early medieval Coptic sources, and even earlier evidence from Pompeii shows its remarkable longevity and adaptability.[8] Despite this widespread diffusion, such formulas were gradually suppressed in later Salernitan manuscript traditions, while reappearing elsewhere in explicitly Christianised forms.[9] This transformation is evident in a range of twelfth- and thirteenth-century manuscripts, including the Rotulus von Mülinen, a codex now preserved at the Österreichische Nationalbibliothek (Cod. 2532), and an English manuscript held by the British Library (Sloane 431).[10] In these cases, Christ is invoked as the agent assisting the woman during childbirth, and the formula is reframed within an overtly devotional context.

By contrast, the *Trotula* version requires the woman to ingest – and thus internalise – the ancient *sator arepo* formula. While the initial cross nominally Christianises the inscription, the formula remains fundamentally pre-Christian in origin. Its efficacy was likely enhanced not only by the act of ingestion but also by its perceived antiquity, which conferred a particular authority upon the written words.[11] As with other graphophagic practices examined in this

8 On the palindrome, see Ernst Darmstaedter, "Die Sator-Arepo-Formel und ihre Erklarung," *Isis* 18 (1932): 322–29; Richard E. Bader, "Sator Arepo: Magik in der Volksmedizin," *Medizinhistorisches Journal* 22 (1987): 115–34. See also William D. Paden and Frances Freeman Paden, "Swollen Woman, Shifting Canon: A Midwife's Charm and the Birth of Secular Romance Lyric," *Publications of the Modern Language Association* 125, no. 2 (2010): 306–21.

9 Green, ed., *The* Trotula, 236, n. 50.

10 Bern, Burgerbibliothek, Cod. 803, fol. 1v: "Ad partu*m* mulieris. Scribe in pane istud carmen. + Adam. + Ada*m*. + Ada*m*. + ueni foras. + Christus te uocat. + S*anct*a maria libera ancilla*m* tua*m* N. Ex ore infantiu*m* et lactentiu*m* d*eu*s p*er*fecisti laude*m* p*ropter* inimicos tuos ut destruas ultore*m* et reuiuiscat infans et da ei ipsu*m* pane manducare et liberabit*ur*. Christus + pax + Christus + pax + Christus + pax + Christus in utero +"; Vienna, Österreichische Nationalbibliothek, Cod. 2532, fols. 125r–v: "Ad partum mulieris. Scribe in pane istud carmen. + Adam + Adam + Adam + ueni foras. + Christus te uocat. + Sancta Maria, libera ancillam tuam N. Ex ore infantium et lactentium perfecisti laudem propter nomen tuum, ut destruas inimicum et reuiuiscat infans. Et da ei ipsum panem manducare, liberabitur." And: "Ad partum. + Christus + pax + Christus + pax + Christus + pax + Christus in utero +. Accipe diptanum et cinamomum et semen aneti et tritum da ei in calido vino bibere; iuuat." On this, see Franz, *Die kirchlichen Benediktionen*, ii, 201–2; London, British Library, Sloane MS 431, fol. 44r: "Si mulier no*n* potest pare. scribe i*n* caseo yel butiro ⁊ da ei manducare *christus* fuit nat*us* de uirgine Maria. ⁊ Ioha*nne*s de elisabeth. adiuro te infans p*er* patrem ⁊ filium ⁊ spiritum sa*nctu*m si puer es an puella: *christus* te appellat foras."

11 Marianne Elsakkers, "In Pain You Shall Bear Children (Gen 3:16): Medieval Prayers for a Safe Delivery," in *Women and Miracle Stories. A Multidisciplinary Exploration*, ed. Anne-Marie Korte (Brill, 2004), 179–209, esp. 195; Frankfurter, "Narrating Power."

book, the power of the remedy did not depend on the patient's comprehension of the text. On the contrary, the opacity of the formula, combined with its physical incorporation into the body, reinforced its perceived potency – especially in contexts where writing itself was understood as a privileged and efficacious medium.

The second remedy preserved in the *Liber de sinthomatibus mulierum* prescribes a drink prepared with another woman's breast milk together with a sequence of letters that does not appear in the earliest version of the text.[12] As in several similar cases discussed earlier, it seems fair to assume that practitioners were expected to know exactly how and where these letters were to be inscribed, to the extent that no further instructions were deemed necessary. If we consider the parallel example found in Sloane 475, they may have been written on the inside of the cup containing the milk with some substance and then dissolved, or directly carved into the cup's interior.[13]

As in the *sator-arepo* formula, such letter-sequences begin to appear only in the earlier witnesses of the *Trotula* proto-ensemble. Charms of this type were hardly characteristic of the Salernitan tradition as a whole. Two notable exceptions, however, occur in the *De aegritudinum curatione tractatus*, a treatise transmitting the work of seven physicians associated with the Salernitan School. Once again, the first of these remedies addresses difficulty in childbirth and recommends writing the phrase *Mentem sanctam, spontaneum humorem domino, et patienti liberationem* on the crust of a loaf of bread.[14] The other remedy is an antidote to snake venom and reads: "When you are informed that someone has been bitten by a serpent or the like, make the messenger stand in the place where they were and turn the right hem of their shirt." A spoonful of water is then poured into a cup three times, and at each pouring the practitioner recites the formula *cara, caruce, senael, emmanuel, paraclitus, in nomine patris et filii et spiritus sancti, amen*, and the Pater Noster. Finally, the patient – or, if absent, the messenger acting as proxy – is to drink the prepared liquid.[15] A

12 In that version, the woman was simply to drink another woman's milk mixed with oil: "bibat lac muliebre cum oleo et statim pariet."

13 London, British Library, Sloane MS 475, fol. 23r.

14 *De aegritudinum curatione tractatus*, in *Collectio salernitana, ossia Documenti inediti, e trattati di medicina appartenenti alla Scuola medica salernitana*, ed. Salvatore De Renzi, 5 vols. (Dalla tipografia del Filiatre-Sebezio, 1852–59), ii, 81–386, at 346: "Ad difficultatem partus scribe hanc scripturam in crusta panis: 'Mentem sanctam, spontaneum humorem domino, et patienti liberationem.'"

15 Ibid., 382: "Cum tibi nuntiatum fuerit aliquem morsum esse a serpente vel hujusmodi, fac nuntium stare in loquo in quo erat et verte dextrum gremium camisie et infunde coclear I. aque, post tria, et post singula trium infundendo dic: 'cara, caruce, senael, emmanuel,

fragment of this formula (*caru. ca*) also appears in an eleventh-century invocation to St. Brendan used to cure snakebite,[16] suggesting that similar sequences of words circulated widely across different textual and devotional contexts.

The symbolic emphasis on the right side in this ritual is consistent with broader medieval associations of the right with positive outcomes and efficacy, as attested, for example, in an original ritual described in Burchard's *Corrector*, compiled around 1010 AD.[17] By contrast, the rationale underlying the choice of particular foods or drinks for specific ailments is less readily recoverable. While some scholars have suggested that certain edible surfaces recur in relation to particular conditions – sacramental wafers (and later sage leaves) for fever, cheese and butter for childbirth[18] – the evidence remains uneven. In the present case, it is more productive to focus on the shared features of these remedies: they are few in number, their texts are believed to exert a direct effect upon reality, and they embody a synthesis of diverse intellectual and cultural traditions.

Equally revealing are the purposes these remedies serve. Treatments for snakebites have a long history, extending back to Graeco-Roman medical literature, and reflect enduring concern over sudden and potentially fatal accidents, much as in the case of rabies.[19] Childbirth, in turn, represented an intensely dramatic and anxiety-laden moment, one that demanded exceptional care and, at times, recourse to verbal formulae and clerical assistance.[20] Just as animal venom threatened life, so the failure of childbirth endangered both

---

paraclitus, in nomine patris et filii et spiritus sancti, amen' et Pater noster, et aquam illam da in potu nuntio vel ipsi patienti si sit presens."

16 Florence, Biblioteca Medicea Laurenziana, Plut. XVII, dext. cod. 12, f. 165v. See Mario Esposito, "Sur la 'Navigatio Sancti Brendani' et sur ses versions italiennes : I. – La *Navigatio*," *Romania* 64, no. 255 (1938): 328–46, at 341.

17 Robert Hertz, "The pre-eminence of the right hand: A study in religious polarity," trans. Rodney and Claudia Needham, *HAU: Journal of Ethnographic Theory* 3, no. 2 (2013): 335–57; Andrea Maraschi, "*Physis* e *Sympatheia*. Un corteo simpatetico femminile per invocare la pioggia nella Renania dell'anno 1000," in *"Con tuono, lampo o pioggia." Magia e stregoneria tempestarie fra antichità ed età moderna*, ed. Vincenzo Tedesco (La Vela, 2023), 87–126, at 96–7.

18 Hindley, *Textual Magic*, 249.

19 Kathleen Walker-Meikle, "Toxicology and Treatment: Medical Authorities and Snake-Bite in the Middle Ages," *Korot – The Israel Journal of the History of Medicine and Science* 22 (2014): 85–104.

20 Valerie French, "Midwives and Maternity Care in the Greco-Roman World," *Helios* 13, no. 2 (1987): 69–84; Paula M. Reider, "Pregnancy and Childbirth: Christian Women," in *Women and Gender in Medieval Europe: An Encyclopedia*, ed. Margaret Schaus (Routledge, 2006), 666–68; Alessandra Foscati, "La scena del parto. Nascita del corpo e salvezza dell'anima tra religione, medicina e 'magia' nell'altomedioevo," in *La presenza dei bambini nelle*

mother and child, thereby justifying the mobilisation of particularly potent remedies, including edible *carmina*.

Given the wide distribution of the *Trotula* corpus, such graphophagic prescriptions became accessible to a broad audience and contributed to the circulation of practices that were by no means confined to the Latin West.[21] While this book has not examined the eastern Mediterranean in detail – apart from brief comparative references – this was a deliberate methodological choice, motivated by my greater familiarity with western and northern European cultures and by the aim of establishing a focused foundation for the study. Nonetheless, it is clear that graphophagy was also practised in the Byzantine world.[22] There, it could function not only as a concrete practice but also as a powerful metaphor.

As shown by manuscript representations of the biblical scenes in Ezekiel and Revelation, the motif of ingesting a written scroll carried rich symbolic meaning. An interesting example is found in the late tenth-century *Menologion* of Basil II, preserved in the Biblioteca Apostolica Vaticana, where the above cited Romanos Melodos is depicted receiving and consuming a scroll offered by the Virgin Mary, thereby being invested with the gift of Christian poetry (fig. 16). This image recalls the account of Cædmon's miraculous acquisition of poetic skill and ultimately derives from the biblical motif of the ingested scroll, underscoring once more the enduring association between internalised text and transformative authority.

Legend has it that, on a Christmas eve around the year 518 Romanos was assigned to read verses from the Psalter while serving in the Church of St. Mary at Blachernae in Constantinople. His performance was so poor that he was immediately replaced by another reader. Ashamed and distressed, Romanos withdrew to the choir stalls, where he fell asleep. The Virgin Mary appeared to him in a dream and handed him a papyrus scroll, inviting him to swallow it. Upon eating the scroll, Romanos awoke to discover that he had acquired extraordinary abilities as a singer and hymnographer.[23]

This story, which presents inspiration as the literal ingestion of text, proved deeply influential and generated a wider literary *topos* of authorial

religioni del Mediterraneo antico: la vita e la morte, i rituali e i culti tra archeologia, antropologia e storia delle religioni, ed. Chiara Terranova (Aracne, 2014), 311–37.

21 Jones and Olsan, "Performative Rituals for Conception," 409.

22 Filippo Ronconi and Stratis Papaioannou, "Book Culture," in *The Oxford Handbook of Byzantine Literature* (Oxford University Press, 2021), 44–75, at 64.

23 José Grosdidier de Matons, *Romanos le Mélode et les origines de la poésie religieuse à Byzance* (Beauchesne, 1977), 162.

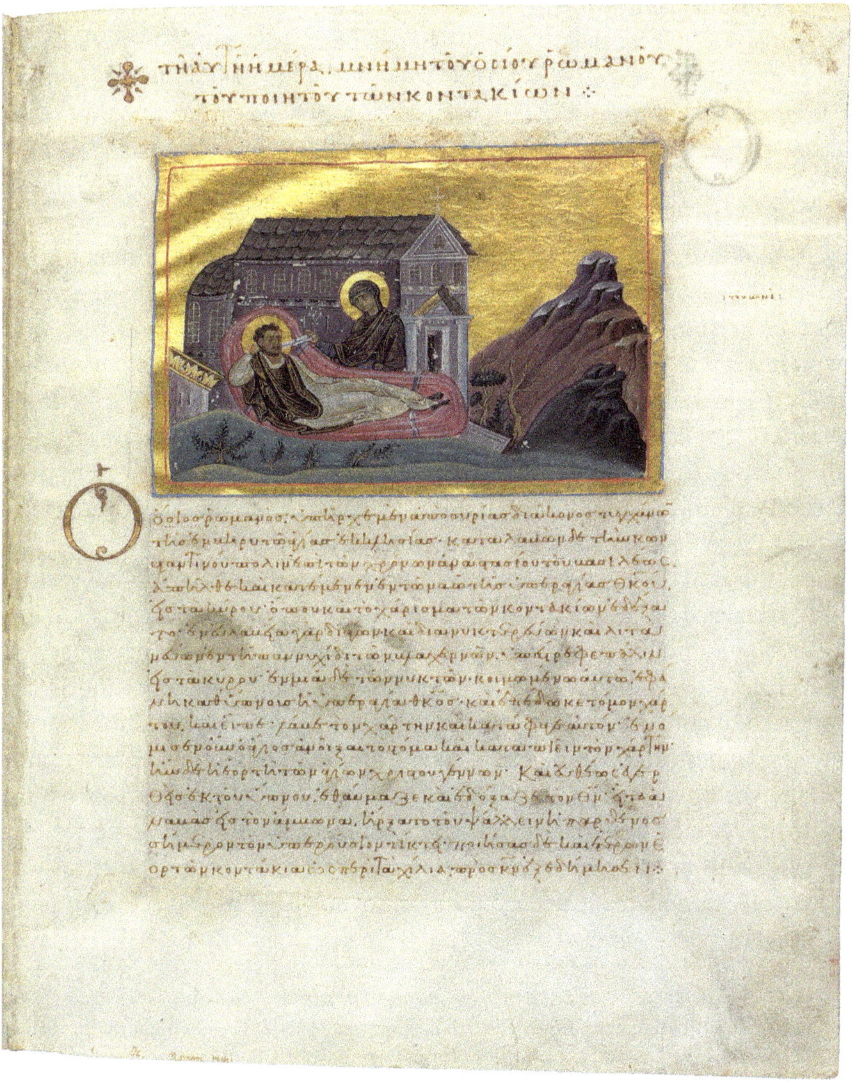

FIGURE 16 Depiction of Romanos the Melodos, eminent 6th-century hymnographer. *Menologion of Basil II*, tenth century, Constantinople. Vatican City, Biblioteca Apostolica Vaticana, Vat. Gr. 1613, fol. 78 (Courtesy of Biblioteca Apostolica Vaticana)

empowerment through graphophagy.[24] A comparable narrative appears, for instance, in the late eleventh-century *Life of Joseph the Hymnographer* by

24 Stratis Papaioannou, "Authors," in *The Oxford Handbook of Byzantine Literature*, 483–524, at 489.

Johannes Galenus, in which the ninth-century Greek monk Joseph similarly consumes a scroll received from the hands of St. Nikolaos.[25] In both cases, poetic and theological authority is represented not as the product of gradual training alone, but as a sudden transformation effected through the internalisation of written words.

In Byzantium, graphophagy was also employed in pedagogical contexts, particularly in the teaching of reading and writing, as discussed above with regard to edible alphabets. In this case, however, the practice does not seem to have relied primarily on familiarity with letters as such. Rather, it drew upon the presumed efficacy of writing materials and the words inscribed upon them. Instead of alphabetic sequences, the names of fantastic or personified angels – Didaktikos ("He who can teach"), Koryphoblepōn ("He who gazes upwards"), Sophotatōs ("The Wisest") – were written on the interior or exterior of vessels into which wine or water was poured. These vessels were then placed beneath the altar during the liturgy, after which the liquid was given to children to drink.[26] Literacy instruction, in this context, was thus assisted by supernatural means, predicated on the internalisation of names associated with specialised entities endowed with cognitive or spiritual authority.

This should not be surprising, as similar practices were widespread across other regions of the Middle East. As noted earlier with reference to the Syrian bowl used to cure rabies, so-called "incantation bowls" circulated extensively between Upper Mesopotamia and Syria from late antiquity until the eighth century. These bowls, typically inscribed in Jewish Babylonian Aramaic within Jewish milieux or in Syriac in Christian contexts, were designed to protect individuals from malevolent forces.[27] Although their primary function was apotropaic rather than pedagogical, they nonetheless reflect the same

25 Johannes Galenus, *Vita S. Josephi*, in *Patrologiae cursus completus, series Graeca*, ed. Jacques-Paul Migne, 105 (Garniers, 1862), 939–75, at 959: "'… Te autem oportet in regiam civitatem contendere, ut confirmes plurimos gratia tibi a Spiritu sancto concessa. Sed prius accipe hoc capitulum, et comede illud.' Videbatur autem habere in dextera exiguum quemdam libellum. Hic vero scripturae quidem illius venustate delectabatur : ea vero, quae ibi scripta erant, interiori animae gutture suavissime recitabat. Erant autem in eo libello scripta haec verba: 'Accelera tanquam misericors, et festina tanquam miserator in adjutorium nostrum: potes enim, si vis.' Et ubi jussus a divino illo viro cecinisset haec cum summa dulcedine ac suavitate, aspexit scripsum a compedibus solutum …"

26 Afanasiĭ Vassiliev, *Anecdota Graeco-Byzantina* (Universitatis Caesareae, 1893), 342; Robert Browning, "Literacy in the Byzantine World," *Byzantine and Modern Greek Studies* 4 (1978): 39–54, at 51–2; repr. in Robert Browning, *History, Language and Literacy in the Byzantine World* (Variorum Reprints, 1989); Guglielmo Cavallo, *Lire a Byzance* (Les belles lettres, 2006), 26–7.

27 Marina Montesano, *Ars Magica. Una storia in 20 oggetti* (Carocci, 2025), 131–37.

underlying assumptions that inform graphophagic practices: that writing possesses inherent efficacy, and that bringing inscribed words into close physical – and at times internal – contact with the body could confer protection, knowledge, or transformation.

Israel Abrahams observed that Jewish children in the medieval period were taught to read by being made to eat letters written with honey: "and the child lisped the letters as he ate the honey, the cakes, and the other delicacies, that the words of the Law might be sweet in his lips."[28] Sometimes, angels were invoked to assist children in the process of learning. Similar pedagogical customs are attested in Coptic Egypt, where they continued even after the Muslims conquest. Coptic grimoires recommend carving powerful words onto wooden boards, rubbing them with lemon, and washing the inscriptions away with water to be drunk. Other times, words were written in honey on alabaster tablets and then diluted in white wine.[29] A sixth- or seventh-century Coptic papyrus now preserved in Cologne records an invocation to the Sun as it rises over Egypt, intended to secure empowerment and protection, and prescribes writing words directly onto the tongue with a pen dipped in black ink.[30]

In later Islamic contexts, Qu'ranic verses were similarly worn or ingested on account of their ritual efficacy, shedding light on the material understanding of the sacred text. This development is particularly striking in light of older and deeply rooted traditions – both in rabbinic Judaism and in Vedic culture – that associated writing with impurity.[31] From the eight century onwards, however, the Qu'ran increasingly came to be treated as a physical object of veneration. The ink used to write Qu'ranic verses was believed to possess healing properties, and according to the scholar Ibn Qayyim al-Jawziyya (1292–1350), written

28 Israel Abrahams, *Jewish Life in the Middle Ages* (Macmillan, 1896), 348.

29 Michael Green, "A Late Coptic Magical Text from the Collection of the Rijksmuseum van Oudheden, Leiden," *Oudheidkundige Mededelingen* 67 (1987): 29–43, esp. 35ff.; Georg Wöhrle, "Papyrophagie," in *"... vor dem Papyrus sind alle gleich!". Papyrologische Beiträge zu Ehren von Bärbel Kramer (P. Kramer)*, ed. Eberhard Raimar, Holger Kockelman, Stefan Pfeiffer, and Maren Schentuleit (de Gruyter, 2009), 243–47.

30 Cologne, Papyrussammlung, P. 20826, fol. 1r. Transcribed in *Ancient Christian Magic*, 110ff.

31 HadžiMuhamedović, "My Grandmother Drank the Qur'an;" Zadeh, "Touching and Ingesting," esp. 461–2. See also Abdullahi Osman El-Tom, "Drinking the Koran: The Meaning of Koranic Verses in Berti Erasure," *Africa: Journal of the International African Institute* 55, 4 (1985): 414–31; Michael Lambek, "Certain Knowledge, Contestable Authority: Power and Practice on the Islamic Periphery," *American Ethnologist*. 17, no. 1 (1990): 23–40; Rudolph T. Ware III, *The Walking Qur'an: Islamic Education, Embodied Knowledge, and History in West Africa* (The University of North Carolina Press, 2014); Hanna Nieber, "'They All Just Want to Get Healthy!' Drinking the Qur'an between Forming Religious and Medical Subjectivities in Zanzibar," *Journal of Material Culture* 22, no. 4 (2017): 453–75.

passages could be immersed in water and drunk as a remedy against the evil eye or to assist women in childbirth.[32] Verses were also inscribed directly onto vessels so that their potency could be transferred to the liquids they contained, or written in saffron ink, which was then dissolved in water. By the eleventh century, scholars attest that Qu'ranic passages were even written onto foods such as sweets, to allow the eater to benefit from the supernatural qualities of the sacred text.

In this respect, the Qu'ran, much like the Bible, was seen as a form of potent medicine – not only in a metaphorical or spiritual sense, but in a practical and embodied one. It therefore seemed natural to mobilise scripture therapeutically. At the same time, such practices raised concerns about the pollution of Qu'ranic verses once ingested as they flowed through the digestive system. These techniques, which predated Islam, required careful adaptation within an Islamic framework. Nonetheless, practice and tradition ultimately prevailed over juridical anxieties, and devotional uses of scripture survived despite periodical legal controversy.[33] By the twelfth century, the inscription of Qu'ranic formulas on the interior surfaces of ceramic bowls had become sufficiently normalised to support specialised production in Egypt and Syria, including brass and bronze vessels.[34] These bowls frequently combine text with talismanic imagery and apotropaic motifs. While sacred text was the subject of sustained juridical debate and figural imagery often remained theologically ambiguous, such objects reveal the convergence of two embodied ritual strategies: iconophagy and graphophagy.

Similar practices are also attested in Christian Nubia, as demonstrated by both archaeological finds and written sources.[35] Their popularity reflect a widespread devotional impulse not merely to imitate sacred figures or texts, but to *become* them – to internalise and appropriate their power. This logic closely parallels the use of early medieval *eulogiae*,[36] whose efficacy depended on physical incorporation rather than symbolic reference alone. As Finbarr Barry Flood has observed, religious rituals across cultures have repeatedly expressed a desire to imbibe, ingest, and incorporate sacred matter, even when

---

32 Ibn Qayyim al-Jawziyya, *Medicine of the Prophet*, trans. Penelope Johnson (Islamic Texts Society, 1998), 128; Zadeh, "Touching and Ingesting," 464.

33 Zadeh, "Touching and Ingesting," 465–6.

34 Flood, "Bodies and Becoming," 477. See also M. Djerbi, "L'incantation mythique : noms et écriture," *Ethnologie française* 23, no. 1 (1993): 94–103; Constant Hamès, ed., *Coran et talismans. Textes et pratiques magiques en milieux musulman* (Karhthala, 2007).

35 Tsakos, "Materiality and Physicality of Medieval Manuscripts," 980–1.

36 Flood, "Bodies and Becoming," 463.

such practices lay at the margins of normative devotion.[37] That these embodied strategies have received relatively little scholarly attention only underscores the importance of recovering graphophagy as a meaningful, if marginal, dimension of premodern religious experience.

Graphophagy is also attested in the influential manual of natural magic and natural philosophy known as *Ghāyat al-hakīm* ("The Goal of the Wise"), written by Maslama b. Qāsim al-Qurṭubī between *c.*954 and 959 and later translated into Castilian and Latin at the court of Alfonso X the Wise under the title *Picatrix*.[38] The author's deliberate anonymity – likely motivated by the controversial nature of the work – already signals the perceived risks associated with its content.[39] The Latin version, while shorter than the Arabic original, incorporates several interpolations.[40]

The *Ghāyat* presents what it terms *siḥr* (rendered as *nigromancia* in Latin, and commonly translated as "magic") not as illicit practice but as a form of natural knowledge embedded within the structure of the cosmos. Although the terminology itself carried ambivalent or negative connotations, the text frames this knowledge as a noble discipline, accessible only to the learned

---

37 Ibid., 461–2.

38 On this text, see: Maribel Fierro, "Bāṭinism in al-Andalus: Maslama b. Qāsim al-Qurṭubī (d. 353/964), Author of the *Rutbat al- Ḥakīm* and the *Ghāyat al-Ḥakīm* (Picatrix)," *Studia Islamica* 84, no. 2 (1996): 87–112; Godefroid de Callataÿ, "Magia en al-Andalus: *Rasā'il Iḫwān al-Ṣafā', Rutbat al-Ḥakīm y Ġāyat al-Ḥakīm* (*Picatrix*)," *Al-Quanṭara* 34, no. 2 (2013): 297–344; Miquel Forcada, "Astrology in al-Andalus during the Eleventh and Twelfth Centuries: Between Religion and Philosophy," in *From Masha'allah to Kepler: Theory and Practice in Medieval and Renaissance Astrology*, ed. Charles Burnett and Dorian Greenbaum (Sophia Centre Press, 2015), 149–76. See also the introductory essays in: *Picatrix: A Medieval Treatise on Astral Magic*, trans. Dan Attrell and David Porreca (The Pennsylvania University Press, 2019); and in *Picatrix: The Latin Version of the* Ghāyat al-hakīm, ed. David Pingree (The Warburg Institute, 1986). On Alphonso's court and the *Picatrix*, see Alejandro García Avilés, "La magie astrale comme art visuel au XIIIe siècle," in *Images et magie.* Picatrix *entre Orient et Occident*, ed. Jean-Patrice Boudet, Anna Caiozzo, and Nicolas Weill-Parot (Champion, 2011), 95–113; Laura Fernández Fernández, *Arte y ciencia en el* scriptorium *de Alfonso X el Sabio* (Universidad de Sevilla/Cátedra Alfonso X el Sabio, 2013); Charles Burnett, "Thābit ibn Qurra the Ḥarrānian on Taslimans and the Spirits of the Planets," *La Corónica*, 36, no. 1 (2007): 13–40; Peter J. Forshaw, "From Occult Ekphrasis to Magical Art Transforming Text into Talismanic Image in the Scriptorium of Alfonso X," in *Bild und Schrift auf "magischen" Artefakten*, ed. Sarah Kiyanrad, Christoffer Theis, and Laura Willer (de Gruyter, 2018), 15–47, at 17–18 and 38–39.

39 Jean-Patrice Boudet and Jean-Charles Coulon, "La version arabe (*Ghāyat al-ḥakīm*) et la version latine du *Picatrix*. Points communs et divergences," *Cahiers de recherches médiévales et humanistes* 33 (2017): 67–101, esp. 77.

40 Béatrice Bakhouche, Frédéric Fauquier, and Brigitte Pérez-Jean, *Picatrix : Un traité de magie médiéval* (Brepols, 2003), 27–28.

and capable of revealing hidden connections between celestial and terrestrial realms.[41] Drawing on a wide range of traditions – Sabian, Babylonian, Egyptian, Indian, Zoroastrian, Greek, Aristotelian, Pythagorean, and Platonic[42] – the work articulates a vision of the universe as a hierarchically ordered system governed by sympathetic correspondences.[43] Within this framework, words and images are endowed with intrinsic efficacy, capable of activating cosmic forces when correctly deployed.[44]

The inclusion of graphophagic rituals in the *Ghāyat* confirms that the ingestion of inscribed matter could be accommodated within learned cosmological systems as well as within vernacular or devotional contexts. In this respect, the *Ghāyat* aligns closely with the theoretical assumption of the treatise *De radiis stellarum*, with its synthesis of Aristotelian and Neoplatonic thought and its emphasis on the material transmission of celestial influence.[45]

In purely Neoplatonic fashion, the *Ghāyat* presents words and signs as essential instruments for activating the forces that permeate the fabric of the universe. Yet prescriptions of graphophagy are rare, a fact that confirms the broader pattern identified throughout this study. In one interpolation absent from the Arabic original and therefore almost certainly introduced at Alphonso's *scriptorium*, the Latin *Picatrix* records two remedies that rely on graphophagic principles. The first addresses the sting of a scorpion, a concern

41 Toufic Fahd, "Siḥr," in *Encyclopaedia of Islam, Second Edition*, ed. Peri Bearman, C. Edmund Bosworth, Edmund van Donzel et al.: http://dx.doi.org/10.1163/1573-3912_islam_SIM_7023; Boudet and Coulon, "La version arabe," 80–82; Fanger, "For Magic," 29. In the Arabic version there also appears the word *nīranj*, from the Persian *nayrang*. Noah Gardiner, "Books on Occult Sciences," in *Treasures of Knowledge: An Inventory of the Ottoman Palace Library (1502/3–1503/4). Volume I: Essays*, ed. Gülru Necipoğlu, Cemal Kafadar, and Cornell H. Fleischer (Brill, 2019), 735–65, at 744; Charles Burnett, "*Nīrānj*, a Category of Magic (almost) Forgotten in the Latin West," in *Natura, scienze e società medievali: Studi in onore di Agostino Paravicini Bagliani*, ed. Claudio Leonardi and Francesco Santi (SISMEL – Edizioni del Galluzzo, 2008), 37–66. On issues concerning the translation into Latin, see Charles Burnett, "Magic in the Court of Alfonso el Sabio: The Latin Translation of the *Ġāyat al-Ḥakīm*," in *De Frédéric II à Rodolphe II. Astrologie, divination et magie dans les cours (XIIIe–XVIIe siècle)*, ed. Jean-Patrice Boudet, Martine Ostorero, and Agostino Paravicini Bagliani (SISMEL – Edizioni del Galluzzo, 2017), 37–52.

42 Willy Hartner, "Notes on Picatrix," *Isis* 56, no. 4 (1965): 438–51. See also Charles Burnett, "East (and South) Asian Traditions in Astrology and Divination as Viewed from the West," *Extrême-Orient Extrême-Occident* 35 (2013): 285–93; Liana Saif, *The Arabic Influences on Early Modern Occult Philosophy* (Palgrave MacMillan, 2015), 37; David Pingree, "Some of the Sources of the Ghāyat al-hakīm," *Journal of the Warburg and Courtauld Institutes* 43 (1980): 1–15, at 2–3.

43 *Picatrix: A Medieval Treatise*, 13.

44 Plotino, *Enneadi*, IV.4.40, 535–50.

45 al-Kindi, *De radiis*, 20.

that reflects the treatise's particular attention to small venomous creatures commonly encountered in urban environments. The antidote involved inscribing a series of names onto a tin tablet and immersing it in water so that the liquid might absorb the words' curative efficacy.[46] If a tin tablet was unavailable, the same names were to be written on the interior of a transparent bowl using an ingestible pigment – such as saffron or a similar substance – after which the bowl was washed with water and the resulting liquid administered to the patient.[47] In keeping with the logic of sympathetic correspondences that underpins the text, the remedy was expected to take effect immediately.[48] The names to write are

> ZAARE ZAARE RAAM ZAARE ZAARE
> FEGEM BOHORIM BORAYN NESFIS ALBUNE
> FEDRAZA AFFETIHE TAUTUTA TANYN ZABAHAT
> AYLATRICYN HAURANE RAHANNIE AYN LATUMINE
> QUEUE ACATYERY NIMIERI QUIBARI YEHUYHA
> NUYYM LATRITYN HAMTAUERY VUERYN
> CATUHE CAHUENE CENHE BEYNE,

followed by Solomon's seal – that is, the Star of David.[49] The sequence of names was arranged in seven lines written on specific days. The instructions emphasise the necessity of absolute accuracy in transcription: any error would compromise the efficacy of the remedy. Such insistence on precision reinforces the idea that power was thought to reside in the correct material configuration of letters and signs, rather than inn their semantic intelligibility. As argued by David Frankfurter, ritual uses of writing in antiquity treated letters and words as materially efficacious substances rather than carriers of meaning.[50] It has been suggested that these names may echo the *Mahāmantra* known from the Sanskrit text *Kali-Saṇṭāraṇa Upaniṣad*, a hypothesis that, while necessarily

46 *Picatrix: The Latin Version of the* Ghāyat al-hakīm, i.5.26, 20: "Et dixit quidam qui semper laboravit ad predicta probandum et istas sciencias, qui venit de terra Nigrorum, qui probavit scribere unum nomen in tabula latonis ipsamque tenebat cu meo. Et quando aliquis percuciebatur a scorpione, lavabat ipsam tabulam in aqua et ipsam dabat percusso in potu; et statim sanabaturm et sedebatur dolor."

47 Ibidem: "Dixit eciam ipse quod quando deficiebat ei tabula latonis, scribebat nomina in scutella limpida cum creta qua scribi poterat quemadmodum crocus et similia que possunt bibi. Et lavabat eam cum aqua et dabat in potu infirmo; et statim dolor cessabat."

48 Schliesser, "Introduction: On Sympathy," 7.

49 *Picatrix: The Latin Version of the* Ghāyat al-hakīm, i.5.27, 20–1.

50 Frankfurter, "The Magic of Writing."

speculative, would point to the extraordinary geographical and intellectual reach of the traditions upon which the *Picatrix* drew.[51] The inclusion of Solomon's seal further situates the remedy within a shared symbolic repertoire that spanned Jewish, Islamic, and Latin learned cultures. In medieval mystical and occult traditions, Solomon's legendary signet was believed to confer authority over spirits and demons, thus reinforcing the protective and coercive dimensions of the prescription. These elements show how graphophagy, though exceptional, could be fully integrated into sophisticated cosmological systems in which writing was understood as a vehicle for transmitting celestial, natural, and supernatural power.

It must be borne in mind that the ultimate goal of the *Ghāyat/Picatrix* was to instruct the aspiring philosopher in the art of *confundere universum* – that is, in mastering the forces that structure the cosmos.[52] The knowledge transmitted by the treatise, and the purposes it was intended to serve, therefore reflect the ambitions of a "wise" man, conceived as an elite figure endowed with exceptional intellectual and technical competence. The form of natural magic described in the text presupposed advanced education, familiarity with cosmological principles, and, not least, expertise in numerological theory. A revealing example appears in a bonding recipe attributed to an Indian king named Behentater – in the Arabic version identified as the physician Kankah al-Hindī.[53] Here, the desired bond between two individuals is effected through the ingestion of specific numbers, administered in food or drink: 220 and 284.[54] These constitute the smallest pair of amicable numbers, each being the sum of the proper divisors of the other. The concept had been known since antiquity and was later the subject of extensive investigation in Islamic mathematics. Because of their intrinsic numerical relationship, these figures were associated with harmony, reciprocity, friendship, and love, and were considered particularly suited to talismanic and ritual applications.[55]

---

51 John M. Greer and Christopher Warnock, *The Picatrix: Liber Rubeus Edition* (Adocentyn Press, 2011), 67.

52 *Picatrix: The Latin Version of the* Ghāyat al-hakīm, Prologue, 3, 1–2.

53 On his identity see Hellmut Ritter and Martin Plessner, *"Picatrix:" Das Ziel des Weisen von Mağrīṭī* (Warburg Institute, 1962), 285–6; Boudet and Coulon, "La version arabe," 70.

54 This remedy has an earlier parallel in both the Arabic and Latin version, which recommends writing the same numbers on two images, which were then to be joined in an embrace. *Picatrix: The Latin Version of the* Ghāyat al-hakīm, i.5.6, 16; *Picatrix, Ghayat al-Hakim, The Goal of the Wise*, I, 39. Another Arabic version of this remedy, which is essentially identical, is in ibid., II, 149–50.

55 Oliver Kahl and Zeina Matar, "A Treatise on the Amicable Numbers 220 and 284 Attributed to Abū Maʿshar al-Balkhī," *Journal of Semitic Studies* 35, no. 2 (1990): 233–43; Roshdi Rashed and Christian Houzel, "Théorie des nombres amiables," in *Thābit ibn Qurra.*

In a closely related procedure intended to induce love, the same numbers were to be carved into a piece of wood and used as a seal to imprint bread dough or other edible substances. The client was instructed to ingest the number 284, while the desired partner consumed 220.[56] Through sympathetic correspondence, the latter was thereby rendered obedient to the former. What is especially noteworthy is the clarification that the efficacy of the operation did not reside *per figuras* – that is, in the written symbols themselves – but *per numerum*, in the numerical value they represented.[57] In other words, the power lay not in the visible signifier, but in the abstract quantity.

This distinction allowed for considerable flexibility in practice. The numbers could be realised through alternative material forms: the client might eat 284 grape or pomegranate seeds, for instance, while the lover-to-be was given 220 of the same fruit. Such instructions underscore the degree to which the *Ghāyat* conceptualised efficacy in terms of numerical essence rather than graphic inscription, while nonetheless preserving a logic of ingestion and internalisation that places these practices directly within a broader graphophagic framework.

Science and Philosophy in Ninth-Century Baghdad, ed. Roshdi Rashed (de Gruyter, 2009), 77–151; Bink Hallum, "New Light on Early Arabic Awfāq Literature," in *Islamicate Occult Sciences in Theory and Practice*, ed. Liana Saif, Francesca Leoni, Matthew Melvin-Koushki, and Farouk Yahya (Brill, 2007), 57–161.

56 *Picatrix: The Latin Version of the* Ghāyat al-hakīm, iii.11.125, 167–8: "Qui vero hunc lapidem primo sua industria compilavit fuit Behentater rex, qui fuit unus ex regibus Indie, sapiens valde. Ipse enim edificavit civitatem de Menif, in qua edificia magna edificavit, et in ipsis edificiis ymagines vociferantes construxit. Hic autem fuit qui invenit computaciones amoris per numerum, quod est unum quid penes eos mirabile valde. He vero computaciones quando [alicui] dantur in cibo vel potu vel alia quacumque re duabus personis, optima coniungentur amicicia et multum ad invicem diligentur. Et si predicti numeri sculpentur in ligno, et cum ipso panem vel aliquid comestibile sigillaveris ipsumque ei dederis comedere, te magno diliget amore. Et si ipsos numeros in tuo signaveris panno, a te non poterit separare [...] Minorque numerus ex ipsis est 220, maior vero numerus est 284. Opus autem predictorum numerorum tale est. Figurabis numerum minorem et maiorem figuris algorismi. Et da minorem cui libuerit in cibo; tu vero maiorem comedas. Ipse vero erit obediens tibi quemadmodum minor est obediens maiori, et diligeris ab eodem propter mirabilem proprietatem et potenciam computacionis predicte."

57 Ibidem: "Hec vero computacio fit similiter in granis passularum et in granis malorum granatorum et in quibuscumque volueris ex fructibus comedendis. Et hoc fit per numerum et non per figuras."

Conclusive Remarks

At this point, it is useful to return to the questions that have guided this study: how, when, and why were graphophagic practices employed, and how significant were they despite their marginality?

At its core, graphophagy rests on the assumption that the efficacy of writing endures beyond the physical presence of the text. When ink was used, most of the time its power derived not from its material composition but from the fact that it had assumed the form of meaningful signs. The sources rarely specify the nature of the ink, implying that efficacy resided primarily in the words themselves. Where signs were written directly onto edible substances, food acquired power through inscription; alternatively, words were understood to transmit their efficacy into food or drink regardless of the material medium.[1] This logic reflects early medieval attitudes towards relics and contact objects: just as matter could be sanctified through proximity to saintly bodies, so words could transfer power to ordinary substances.[2]

This analysis confirms the methodological premise adopted throughout: rather than treating graphophagy as residual magic or irrational survival, it is more productive to understand it as a ritual technique grounded in widely shared assumptions about materiality, transmission, and embodied efficacy. The sources rarely conceptualise these acts as belonging to a distinct category. Their coherence emerges only when examined within immediate cultural, textual, and therapeutic contexts – contexts in which boundaries between medicine, devotion, and what modern readers might call magic remained fluid.

Reconstructing the history of graphophagy in early and high medieval Europe remains necessarily fragmentary. The practice is well attested in late antiquity, where Greco-Roman, Jewish, and early Christian textual cultures converged. Evidence surfaces more sparsely in early medieval Ireland, where Latin learning and vernacular tradition intersected. From the ninth century onward, graphophagy becomes more substantial in the Carolingian world, likely facilitated by Mediterranean textual circulation alongside efforts to regulate vernacular healing practices. By the tenth and eleventh centuries, it is firmly embedded in Anglo-Saxon medical culture, while in Scandinavia it appears

1 Hindley, "Eating Words and Burning Them," 370.

2 E.g.: Raymond Van Dam, *Saints and Their Miracles in Late Antique Gaul* (Princeton University Press, 1993); Freeman, *Holy Bones, Holy Dust*; Gary Vikan, "Ruminations on Edible Icons: Originals and Copies in the Art of Byzantium," *Studies in the History of Art* 20 (1989): 47–59; Robert Wiśniewski, *The Beginnings of the Cult of Relics* (Oxford University Press, 2019).

HTTPS://DOI.ORG/10.1163/9789004765528-008

in mythological narratives and ritual contexts attested by runic inscriptions. From al-Andalus and southern Italy – regions where Arabic, Greek, Latin, and vernacular traditions converged – graphophagy entered learned medical and natural-philosophical discourse. The uneven survival of sources precludes linear continuity, yet the convergence of literary, medical, and material evidence allows graphophagy to be treated as historically relevant rather than a purely literary motif.

The conditions addressed by graphophagic remedies form a coherent cluster. They predominantly concern states of bodily imbalance and internal disruption, including poisoning, haemorrhage, fevers, gastrointestinal disorders, rabies, epilepsy, and complications in childbirth. Additionally, graphophagy addressed conditions at the intersection of body and mind – insomnia, forgetfulness, emotional distress, lovesickness – and served to protect individuals from malevolent entities or invoke divine intervention. These conditions must have required action from within the body rather than external treatment. Last but not least, graphophagy was still employed in Christian contexts as a means for identifying thieves when testimony or clear evidence was lacking.

This internal mode of action sets graphophagy apart from textual amulets, which work through proximity and constant presence, and from spoken charms, which operate through vocalisation and ritual performance. Graphophagy takes things further: it annihilates the boundary between text and body entirely. The word does not merely accompany or protect – it gets absorbed into the person's metabolic and spiritual systems.

Another dimension worth considering is taste and sensory experience. For different reasons, palatability mattered in antiquity and the Middle Ages much as it does today. In antiquity, taste was a key sensory tool for identifying a plant's properties.[3] Bitterness, associated with many medicinal substances, signalled both efficacy and potential toxicity.[4] In Levi-Straussian terms, medicines must therefore be not only "good to think" but also "good to ingest." Graphophagic practices stand out precisely because they involved deliberate consumption of substances that were culturally and sensorially unconventional – blood, ink, dissolved parchment, or inscribed organic matter. In this sense, graphophagy erased conventional boundaries of taste and disgust, redefining what could be rendered edible to pursue aims that went beyond nourishment.

---

3 Laurence B. Totelin, *Taste and the Ancient Senses* (Routledge, 2017).

4 Julie A. Mennella, Alan C. Spector, Danielle R. Reed, and Susan E. Coldwell, "The Bad Taste of Medicines: Overview of Basic Research on Bitter Taste," *Clinical Therapeutics* 35, no. 8 (2013): 1225–46; John N. Coupland and John E. Hayes, "Physical Approaches to Masking Bitter Taste: Lessons from Food and Pharmaceuticals," *Pharmaceutical Research* 31 (2014): 2921–39.

When words were not inscribed directly onto food, various inks could be employed. Descriptions are rare, because efficacy was often thought to reside in the words rather than in the substances used to write them. Sources occasionally mention inks made from ground charcoal or from galls, rich in gallic and tannic acids. These were crushed and mixed with water or wine, later combined with green vitriol and a binder such as gum Arabic.[5] The ingestion of such inks might cause gastrointestinal discomfort or irritation if taken in quantity, yet when consumed occasionally, in small amounts and diluted, side effects would have been minimal. These potential discomforts were evidently considered negligible in cultures that placed their trust in the efficacy of the inscribed signs themselves.

Despite its wide chronological and geographical diffusion, graphophagy remained structurally marginal. This marginality was not accidental but reflects the practice's position at the intersection of multiple conflicting discourses and authorities. The practice presupposed access to writing and often to specialised knowledge – runic, biblical, or formulaic – placing it in an ambiguous space between learned medicine, devotional practice, and vernacular healing. Improper execution could be ineffective at best, or dangerous at worst, contributing to the perception of graphophagy as a practice requiring expertise and restraint rather than routine use. Moreover, this marginality was reinforced by theological anxieties. Early medieval authorities expressed concern about excessive reliance on words detached from proper sacramental or devotional context, fearing such practices might constitute illicit invocation or demonic commerce. Graphophagy occupied precisely the zone of maximum theological anxiety: it involved material destruction of sacred or powerful texts, bodily incorporation of signs, and claims to operative efficacy that bypassed institutional mediation. This may help explain why graphophagic remedies are scattered or appear most often in marginal manuscript spaces rather than in authoritative medical compendia or liturgical books.

Graphophagy must thus be understood within a broader culture of verbal and textual efficacy rather than as an anomalous or purely magical phenomenon. Across the sources examined, words are consistently portrayed as operative when used correctly. Graphophagy represents an intensification of this widely shared assumption: by connecting text and body, the ingestion of writing makes language not merely symbolically but metabolically effective.

5 Thomas Christiansen, "Manufacture of Black Ink in the Ancient Mediterranean," *The Bulletin of the American Society of Papyrologists* 54 (2017): 167–95; Ira Rabin, "Material Studies of Historic Inks: Transition from Carbon to Iron-Gall Inks," in *Traces of Ink. Experiences of Philology and Replication*, ed. Lucia Raggetti (Brill, 2021), 70–8.

Writing, in these contexts, was not a passive representation but an active substance capable of being assimilated and activated within the living body.[6]

This understanding aligns with broader discussions of performativity and cosmic connection. Graphophagic formulae appear to assume that properly formed words participate structurally in cosmic order. This kind of performative efficacy depended on social recognition and institutional backing, though. Graphophagy thus operated within multiple overlapping authority systems: clerical literacy and sacramental power, traditional knowledge passed through familial or local networks, and the inherent authority of ancient or foreign formulae perceived as powerful precisely because of their obscurity or antiquity.

The comparative approach adopted in this book aims at demonstrating that graphophagy was not culturally isolated. While local variations are evident, similar techniques recur across regions and periods. These parallels shed light on shared assumptions about sympathy and embodiment. Over time, the practice did not disappear but adapted to changing cultural and institutional contexts. The consumed texts reveal important continuities, too: short formulae, repetitive sequences, divine names, and sacred verses predominate. Semantic transparency was often subordinate to recognisability, rhythm, visual or acoustic symmetry, antiquity, foreignness, and symbolic authority. Materials were frequently chosen for accessibility and ease of inscription rather than exotic qualities, suggesting that letters were understood as materially potent entities instead of mere vehicles of meaning.

By isolating and analysing graphophagic practices as a coherent phenomenon, this book contributes to ongoing debates on ritual efficacy, the materiality of language, and the permeability of categories such as religion, medicine, and magic in medieval Europe. It shows that practices often dismissed as marginal or irrational were embedded in consistent modes of reasoning and shared cultural logics. Graphophagy's otherness derived not from sheer strangeness but from its liminal position – simultaneously textual and corporeal, learned and vernacular, orthodox and potentially heterodox. Its adaptability reflected the pluralistic nature of medieval healing cultures, in which multiple explanatory frameworks coexisted and practitioners drew pragmatically on whatever resources seemed effective. Its quasi-universality, rooted in analogical reasoning and belief in supernatural agency, helps explain why similar practices appear independently across cultures, yet the specific forms graphophagy took were always dependent on the relative cultural and historical context.

6 Cf. Sophie Page, "Medieval Magic," in *The Oxford History of Witchcraft and Magic*, ed. Owen Davies (Oxford University Press, 2023), 29–61, at 29–32.

Ultimately, graphophagy illustrates how medieval Europeans negotiated anxiety and agency. It represented a coherent response to perceived limits of control and of institutional medicine, to the uncertainties of therapeutic knowledge, and to the existential precariousness of life. Though structurally marginal, graphophagy was thus an enduring strategy within medieval cultures of healing, devotion, and protection. It also offered therapeutic responses for conditions where conventional medicine acknowledged its own limits. In this sense, graphophagy functioned as a ritual technology of last resort – not because it was considered inferior or ineffective, but because it addressed situations of dramatic uncertainty and urgency.

The enduring practice of graphophagy across centuries and diverse therapeutic contexts cannot be attributed to a single cause, but rather to a confluence of factors that sustained its cultural and medical legitimacy. Important among these were the perceived authority of sacred or authoritative texts imbued with power, the trust invested in ritual practitioners or clerical intermediaries, and the habitual reinforcement through repeated communal or individual acts of ingestion, which conferred familiarity and psychological reassurance. Yet one must also take into account the empirical observation of perceived positive responses among those who consumed such texts. In an age when Galenic humoural medicine frequently proved at best innocuous and at worst deleterious, the symbolic ingestion of inscribed words offered a seemingly valid alternative. Contemporary placebo research reveals substantial symptomatic relief – typically ranging from 30–50% improvement – especially for subjective conditions like chronic pain, mood disorders, anxiety, and sensory issues such as persistent cough or eye discomfort. These conditions partially overlap with those traditionally addressed through word consumption. The mechanism behind placebo effects involves expectation, contextual factors, and genuine neurobiological changes in how we perceive and process symptoms.[7]

The history of graphophagy is the history of a largely neglected dimension of medieval textual culture – one in which writing was not only read or heard, but eaten, absorbed, and activated within the body itself. Such practices remind us that, for medieval societies, words were not inert signs but material forces

7 Curtis E. Margo, "The Placebo Effect," *Survey of Ophthalmology* 44, no. 1 (1999): 31–44; Enck Paul and Sibylle Klosterhalfen, "Placebo Responses and Placebo Effects in Functional Gastrointestinal Disorders." *Front Psychiatry* Aug 25, 11, 797 (2020), doi: https://doi.org/10.3389/fpsyt.2020.00797; Giorgos Tzigkounakis, Katerina Simati, Konstantinos Georgiadis, "The Placebo Effect in Medicine and Clinical Practice: A Narrative Review," *Cureus* Sep 9, 17, 9 (2025): e91893, doi: 10.7759/cureus.91893; Mayar B. Alnasralla and Basel H. Nasralla, "Placebo Effects in Modern Medicine: Mechanisms, Clinical Evidence, Limitations, and Future Directions," *Cureus* Jan 2. 18, 1 (2026): e100612, doi: 10.7759/cureus.100612.

capable of acting upon the world. The paradox at the heart of graphophagy – that writing must be destroyed to work – reveals a distinctive understanding of textual efficacy. Unsurprisingly, graphophagy has survived into the present,[8] since human societies have long tried to reach towards natural or supernatural powers in order to effect change in the world.[9]

This book has tried to render visible what has remained conceptually invisible: the consumption of words as a coherent ritual practice with its own internal logic, social functions, and cultural meanings. In doing so, it has necessarily drawn boundaries around a phenomenon that medieval people themselves rarely conceptualised as unified or discrete.

Special words for societies of word eaters.

8 See, for instance: Onésyme Durocher, "De la bibliophagie," in *Miscellanies of the Philobiblon Society* 10 (Whittingham and Wilkins, 1866–67), 195–210; Franz Dornseiff, *Das Alphabet in Mystik und Magie* (Teubner, 1922); Walker, "On Logophagy," 18–9; Pritchard, "On Bibliomancy"; Goody, "Restricted Literacy in Northern Ghana." See also the amulets preserved at the Museum of Ethnomedicine Antonio Scarpa in Genova, Italy: https://www.etnomedicina.unige.it/collezioni/amuleto-e-talismano/.

9 Albrecht Classen, "Magic in the Middle Ages and the Early Modern Age – Literature, Science, Religion, Philosophy, Music, and Art. An Introduction," in *Magic and Magicians in the Middle Ages and the Early Modern Time*, 1–108, at 8.

Bibliography

Primary Sources

a. Manuscripts

ATA, Ämbetsarkiv 2, Vitterhetsakademiens handskriftsamling, serie F 16 v. 26.

Bamberg, Staatsbibliothek, MS Med. 2 (L.III.6).

Bern, Burgerbibliothek, Cod. 803.

Cambridge, Corpus Christi College, MS 391.

Chantilly, Musée Condé, 0599 (1426).

Cologne, Erzbischöfliche Diözesan- und Dombibliothek, Cod. 198.

Cologne, Papyrussammlung, P. 20826.

Dijon, Bibliothèque Municipale, MS 448.

Dublin, RIA MS 24 B 3, 92–93.

Dublin, Trinity College MS 57 (*Book of Durrow*).

Einsiedeln, Stiftsbibliotheck MS 281.

Exeter, Cathedral Library 3501.

Florence, Biblioteca Medicea Laurenziana, Plut. XVII, dext. cod. 12.

Laon, Bibliothèque municipal, MS 420.

Leiden, Universiteitsbibliotheek MS BPL 126.

Leiden, Universiteitsbibliotheek MS VLF 74.

London, British Library, Egerton MS 821.

London, British Library, Harley MS 585.

London, British Library, Royal MS 12 D. xvii.

London, British Library, Add MS 19725.

London, British Library, Egerton MS 833.

London, British Library, Sloane MS 3564.

London, British Library, Sloane MS 431.

London, British Library, Sloane MS 475.

London, Lambeth Palace Library, MS 3.

Los Angeles, Getty Museum, Ludwig III 1 (83.MC.72).

Paris, BNF, MS Latin 16744.

Paris, BNF, MS Latin 6880.

Paris, BNF, MS Latin 229.

St. Gallen, Stiftsbibliothek, Cod. Sang. 44.

St. Gallen, Stiftsbibliothek, 751.

Trier, Stadtbibliothek MS 40/1018.

Uppsala, Universitetsbiblioteket C. 664.

 | HTTPS://DOI.ORG/10.1163/9789004765528-009

Vatican City, Biblioteca Apostolica Vaticana, Barb. lat. 160.
Vatican City, Biblioteca Apostolica Vaticana, Vat. Gr. 1613.
Vienna, Österreichische Nationalbibliothek, Cod. 2532.
Worcester Cathedral Library, Ms Q.5.

b. Edited Sources

Agostino. *La città di Dio*, ed. Luigi Alici. Bompiani, 2001.

Atkinson, Robert, ed. and trans. *The Passions and the Homilies from Leabhar Breac: Text, Translation and Glossary*. Hodges Figgis, 1887.

Augustine of Hippo. *De doctrina christiana*, ed. Joseph Martin, CCSL 32. Brepols, 1962.

Augustine of Hippo. *Sermones ad populum*, in *Sancti Augustini Sermones post Maurinos reperti*, ed. Germain Morin, *Miscellanea Agostiniana*, vol. 1. Tipografia Poliglotta Vaticana, 1930.

Autpert Ambrose. *Expositio in Apocalypsin*, ed. Robert Weber, CCCM 27; 27A. Brepols, 1975.

Bernard, John H., and Robert Atkinson, ed. *Preface to the Hymn of St. Sechnall*, in *The Irish Liber Hymnorum*, 3–13. Harrison and Sons, 1898.

Betha Colaim Chille. Life of Columcille. Compiled by Manus O'Donnell in 1532. Edited and translated from manuscript Rawlinson B. 514 in the Bodleian Library, Oxford, ed. Andrew O'Kelleher and Gertrude Schoepperle. University of Illinois, 1918.

Betz, Hans Dieter, ed. *The Greek Magical Papyri in Translation Including the Demotic Spells*. The University of Chicago Press, 1986.

Biblia Sacra Vulgata. Ed. Robert Weber and Roger Gryson, 5th ed. Deutsche Bibelgesellschaft, 2007.

Bjarni Einarsson, ed. *Egils saga*. Viking Society for Northern Research, 2003.

Bugge, Sophus, and Magnus Olsen. *Norges Indskrifter med de ældre Runer. Inledning*, 3 vols. Brøgger, 1891–1924.

Caesarius of Arles. *Sancti Caesarii Arelatensis Sermones*, ed. Germain Morin, CCSL 103–104. Brepols, 1953.

Caius Julius Solinus. *Collectanea Rerum Memorabilium*, ed. Theodor Mommsen. Weidmann, 1895.

Caspari, Carl P., ed. *Homilia de sacrilegiis*, in *Eine Augustin fälschlich beilegte Homilia de sacrilegiis*. Jacob Dybwad, 1886.

Cockayne, Oswald, ed. and trans. *Leechdoms, Wortcunning, and Starcraft of Early England, Being a Collection of Documents Illustrating the History of Science in this Country Before the Norman Conquest*, 3 vols. Longman, Green, Longman, Roberts, and Green, 1864–66 [repr. Cambridge University Press, 2012].

De aegritudinum curatione tractatus. In *Collectio salernitana, ossia Documenti inediti, e trattati di medicina appartenenti alla Scuola medica salernitana*, 5 vols., ii, 81–386. Dalla tipografia del Filiatre-Sebezio, 1852–59.

De Vriend, Hubert Jan, ed. *The Old English Herbarium and Medicina de Quadrupedibus.* Oxford University Press, 1984.

Deegan, Marilyn, ed. *A Critical Edition of MS.B.L.Royal 12.D.xvii: Bald's Leechbook,* unpub. Ph.D. Diss. University of Manchester, 1988.

Ferraces Rodríguez, Arsenio. "Liber compositionum medicinalium Sangallense-Upsaliensis (= "das St. Galler antidotarium", Sigerist, pp. 78–99)." *Galenos: Rivista di filologia dei testi medici antichi* 15 (2021): 33–58.

Ferraces Rodríguez, Arsenio. "Magia, medicina y veterinaria en la antigüedad tardía. *Editio princeps* del recetario médico *Ad cauculum.*" *Maia* 65, no. 1 (2013): 75–94.

Franz, Adolph. *Die kirchlichen Benediktionen im Mittelalter,* 2 vols. Herdersche Verlagshandlung, 1909 [repr. Akademische Druck und Verlagsanstalt, 1960].

Gerald of Wales. *Topographia Hibernica,* in Id., *Opera,* 8 vols., vol. 5, ed. James F. Dimock. Longmans, Green, Reader, and Dyer, 1867.

Giovanni Boccaccio. *Decameron,* ed. Vittore Branca, 2 vols. Mondadori, 2005 [1985].

Grágás: Islændernes lovbog i fristatens tid, udg. efter det kongelige Bibliotheks Haanskrift, ed. Vilhjálmur Finsen, 2 vols. Odense Universitetsforlag, 1974 [1852].

Green, Monica H., ed. *The* Trotula*: An English Translation of the Medieval Compendium of Women's Medicine.* University of Pennsylvania Press, 2002.

Gregory of Tours. *De passione et virtutibus sancti Juliani martyris,* ed. Bruno Krusch, MGH SSRM 1.2, 112–134. Hahn, 1885.

Gregory of Tours. *De virtutibus sancti Martini episcopi,* ed. Bruno Krusch, MGH SSRM 1.2, 134–211. Hahn, 1885.

Gregory of Tours. *Historiarum libri decem,* ed. Bruno Krusch and Wilhelm Levison, MGH SSRM 1.1. Hahn, 1937–1951.

Gregory the Great. *Homiliae in Hiezechihelem prophetam,* ed. Marcus Adriaen, CCSL 142. Brepols, 1971.

Griffith, Francis L., and Herbert Thompson, ed. *The Demotic Magical Papyrus of London and Leiden.* H. Grevel&Co., 1904.

Guðrúnarkviða II. In *Eddukvæði,* ed. Jónas Kristjánsson and Vésteinn Ólason, 2 vols., II, 352–61. Hið íslenzka bókmenntafélag, 2014.

Hávamál. In *Eddukvæði,* ed. Jónas Kristjánsson and Vésteinn Ólason, 2 vols., II, 322–55. Hið íslenzka bókmenntafélag, 2014.

Horace. *Epistles. Book I,* ed. Roland Mayer. Cambridge University Press, 1994.

Ibn Qayyim al-Jawziyya. *Medicine of the Prophet,* trans. Penelope Johnson. Islamic Texts Society, 1998.

Isidoro di Siviglia. *Etimologie o origini,* ed. Angelo Valastro Canale. Utet, 2013.

Jefford, Clayton N., ed. *Didache. The Teaching of the Twelve Apostles.* Polebridge Press, 2013

Jerome. *Commentariorum in Hiezechielem libri XIV,* ed. Francisco Glorie, CCSL 75, 3–743. Brepols, 1964.

Johannes Galenus. *Vita S. Josephi*, in *Patrologiae cursus completus, series Graeca*, ed. Jacques-Paul Migne, 105, 939–75. Garniers, 1862.

John of Salisbury. *Metalogicon*, ed. John B. Hall and Katharine S.B. Keats-Rohan, CCCM 98. Brepols, 1991.

Jörimann, Julius, ed. *Frühmittelalterliche Rezeptarien*. Orell Fussli, 1925.

Keller, Otto, ed. *Pseudacronis scholia in Horatium vetustiora*, ed., 2 vols. Teubner, 1902–04.

Larrington, Carolyne, trans. "The Lay of Sigrdrifa." In *The Poetic Edda*, 162–8. Oxford University Press, 2014.

Larsen, Henning, ed. *An Old Icelandic Medical Miscellany. MS Royal Irish Academy 23 D 43*. Dybwad, 1931.

Leabhar Breac, the Speckled Book, Otherwise Styled Leabhar M'or D'una Daighre, the Great Book of Dun Doighre; A Collection of Pieces in Irish and Latin, Compiled from Ancient Sources about the Close of the Fourteenth Century, ed. Seosamh Ó Longáin and John J. Gilbert. Royal Irish Academy House, 1872–76.

Lindqvist, Natan, ed. *En isländsk svartkonstbok från 1500-talet* (*Galdrabók*). Appelbergs boktryckeri aktiebolag, 1921.

Macalister, Robert A.S., ed. *The book of Mac Carthaigh Riabhach, otherwise the Book of Lismore*. The Stationery Office, 1950.

Marcellus Empiricus. *De Medicamentis Liber*, ed. Maximilian Niedermann, trans. Jutta Kollesch and Diethard Nickel, 2nd ed. Akademie-Verlag, 1968.

Marsden, Richard. *The Cambridge Old English Reader*. Cambridge University Press, 2004.

Martin, Jean-Pierre Paulin. *Actes du Brigandage d'Ephèse. Traduction faite sur le texte syriaque contenu dans le manuscript 14530 du Musée britannique*. E. Glorieux, 1874.

Martin of Braga. *De correctione rusticorum*. In *Martini Episcopi Bracarensis opera omnia*, ed. Claude W. Barlow. Yale University Press, 1950.

Murphy, Denis, ed. *The Annals of Clonmacknoise, being Annals of Ireland from the Earliest Period to A.D. 1408, translated into English A.D. 1627 by Conell Mageohegan*. Dublin University Press, 1896.

Ordines iudiciorum Dei. In Formulae *Merowingici et Karolini aevi. Ordines iudiciorum Dei*, ed. Karl Zeumer, 599–722. Hahn, 1886.

Paenitentiale Merseburgense a (*recensio W10*). In *Paenitentialia minora Franciae et Italiae*, ed. Raymund Kottje, CCSL 156, 126–64. Brepols, 1994.

Pedanius Dioscorides of Anazarbus. *De materia medica*, trans. Lily Y. Beck. Olms-Weidmann, 2005.

Perosa, Alessandro, ed. *Giovanni Rucellai ed il suo zibaldone. I: 'Il zibaldone quaresimale.'* Warburg Institute, 1960.

Pettit, Edward. *Anglo-Saxon Remedies, Charms, and Prayers from British Library MS Harley 585: The «Lacnunga»*, 2 vols. The Edwin Mellen Press, 2001.

Picatrix, Ghayat al-Hakim, The Goal of the Wise. Trans. From the Arabic by Hashem Atallah, 2 vols. Ouroboros Press, 2002.

Picatrix: A Medieval Treatise on Astral Magic. Trans. Dan Attrell and David Porreca. The Pennsylvania University Press, 2019.

Picatrix: The Latin Version of the Ghāyat al-hakīm. Ed. David Pingree. The Warburg Institute, 1986.

Pliny the Elder. *Naturalis Historia libri XXXVII*, ed. Karl F.T. Mayhoff. Teubner, 1906.

Plotino. *Enneadi*, ed. Giovanni Reale and Roberto Radice. Mondadori, 2008.

Plummer, Charles, ed. and trans. *Life of Brendan of Clonfert*, in *Lives of Irish Saints*, 2 vols., 44–92. Oxford University Press, 1922.

Poenitentiale Valicellanum III. In *Die Bussordnungen der abendländischen Kirche nebst einer rechtsgeschichtlichen Einleitung*, ed. Friedrich Wilhelm Hermann Wasserschleben, 682–88. Ch. Graeger, 1851 [repr. 1958].

Pseudo-Theodorus Priscianus. *Additamenta Pseudo-Theodori ad Theodorum Priscianum*, ed. Valentino Rose. Teubner, 1894.

Quintiliano. *L'istituzione oratoria*, ed. Rino Faranda and Piero Pecchiura. UTET, 2003.

Quinto Orazio Flacco, *Le satire*, in Id., *Le opere*, ed. Tito Colamarino and Domenico Bo. UTET, 2013.

Rabanus Maurus. *De institutione clericorum*, ed. Detlev Zimpel, 2 vols. Brepols, 2006.

Regino of Prüm. *Libri duo de synodalibus causis et disciplinis ecclesiasticis*, ed. Friedrich G.A. Wasserschleben. Akademische Druck- u. Verlagsanstalt, 1964 [1840].

Såby, Viggo, ed. *Det arnamagnæanske handskrift nr. 187 i ocktav, indeholdende en dansk lægebog*. Thieles Bogtrykkeri, 1883.

Saxo Grammaticus. *Gesta Danorum. Danmarkshistorien*, ed. Karsten Friis-Jensen, trans. Peter Zeeberg, 2 vols. Danske Sprog- og Litteraturselskab & Gads Forlag, 2005.

Scandinavian Runic-text Database, Department of Scandinavian Languages, Uppsala University. https://app.raa.se/open/runor/search.

Scudder, Bernard, trans. *Egils Saga*, in *The Complete Sagas of the Icelanders, Including 49 Tales*, ed. Viðar Hreinsson, 5 vols., I, 33–177. Leifur Eiríksson, 1997.

Sigerist, Henry E., ed. *Studien und Texte zur Frühmittelalterlichen Rezeptliteratur*. Verlag von Johann Ambrosius Barth, 1923.

Sigrdrífumál. In *Eddukvæði*, ed. Jónas Kristjánsson and Vésteinn Ólason, 2 vols., II, 313–21. Hið íslenzka bókmenntafélag, 2014.

Skírnismál. In *Eddukvæði*, ed. Jónas Kristjánsson and Vésteinn Ólason, 2 vols., I, 380–88. Hið íslenzka bókmenntafélag, 2014.

Snorri Sturluson, *Ynglinga saga*, in *Heimskringla* I, ed. Bjarni Aðalbjarnarson. Íslenzk fornrít XXVI, 9–83. Hið íslenska bókmenntafélag, 1941.

Stokes, Whitley, ed. "Life of Colomb Cille." In *Lives of saints, from the Book of Lismore*, 168–81. Clarendon, 1890.

Stokes, Whitley, ed. *Three Middle-Irish Homilies on the Lives of Saints Patrick, Brigit and Columba*. Privately printed, 1877.

Stoll, Ulrich, ed. *Das 'Lorscher Arzneibuch'. Ein medizinisches Kompendium des 8. Jahrhunderts (Codex Bambergensis medicinalis 1). Text, Übersetzung und Fachglossar*. Franz Steiner, 1992.

Sudhoff, Karl. "Codex medicus Hertensis (Nr. 192). Handschriftstudie." *Archiv für Geschichte der Medizin* 10, no. 6 (1917): 265–313.

Tesdorpf, Paul, and Therese Tesdorpf-Sickenberger, ed. *Das Medizinische Lehrgedicht der Hohen Schule zu Salerno: Regimen sanitatis Salerni*. Verlag von W. Kolhammer, 1915.

The Cannibal Hymn. In *Writings from Ancient Egypt*, trans. Toby Wilkinson. Penguin, 2016.

Vafþrúðnismál. In *Eddukvæði*, ed. Jónas Kristjánsson and Vésteinn Ólason, 2 vols., I, 356–66. Hið íslenzka bókmenntafélag, 2014.

Van Kirk Dobbie, Elliott, ed. *The Anglo-Saxon Minor Poems*. Columbia University Press, 1942.

Venantius Fortunatus. *Vita Germani Parisiaci* 54, ed. Wilhelm Levison, MGH SSRM 7. Hahn, 1920.

Venerable Bede. *Bede's ecclesiastical history of the English people*, ed. and trans. Beltram Colgrave and R.A.B. Mynors. Clarendon Press, 1969.

Venerable Bede. *Libri quatuor in principium Genesis usque ad nativitatem Isaac et eiectionem Ismahelis adnotationum*, ed. Charles W. Jones, CCSL 118A. Brepols, 1967.

Vogel, Cyrille, and Reinhard Elze, ed. *Le Pontifical romano-germanique du dixième siècle*, 3 vols. Biblioteca Apostolica Vaticana, 1963.

Völsunga saga. In *Fornaldar sögur Norðurlanda*, 4 vols., ed. Guðni Jónsson, I, 107–218. Íslendingasagnaútgáfan, 1954.

Wright, F.A., ed. *Select letters of St. Jerome*. Putnam, 1933.

Ya'Qub Ibn Ishaq al-Kindi. *De radiis. Teorica delle arti magiche. Un trattato medievale di magia naturale e astrologia fondamentale per l'Islam e l'Occidente*, ed. Ezio Abrile and Stefano Fumagalli, trans. Emanuela Turri. Mimesis, 2014 [1994].

Studies

Abrahams, Israel. *Jewish Life in the Middle Ages*. Macmillan, 1896.

Acerbi, Silvia. "Acusaciones de magia contra obispos: el caso de Sofrino de Tella." *Codex Aquilarensis. Cuadernos de investigación del Monasterio de Santa María la Real* 17 (2001): 129–42.

Ager, Britta K. *The Scent of Ancient Magic*. University of Michigan Press, 2022.

Agut-Mabordère, Damien, and Michel Chauveau, ed. *Héros, magiciens et sages oubliés de l'Égypte ancienne: Une anthologie de la littérature en égyptien démotique*. Les Belles Lettres, 2011.

Alexandre-Bidon, Danièle. "Abécédaires et alphabets éducatifs du XIIIe à la fin du XVe siècle." *Nouvelles de l'Estampe* 90 (1986): 6–10.

Alexandre-Bidon, Danièle. "La lettre volée. Apprendre à lire à l'enfant au Moyen Âge." *Annales E.S.C.* 44 (1989): 953–92.

Alexandre-Bidon, Danièle. *Alphabets: 1470–1700 : À lire, à dire, à écrire, à broder*, Catalogue de l'exposition. Paris, Bibliothèque Nationale, Réserve des Livres Rares et Precieux, 1990.

Allen, Ronald B. "Numbers." In *The Expositor's Bible Commentary: Genesis, Exodus, Leviticus, Numbers*, vol. 2, ed. Frank E. Gaebelein, 655–1008. Zondervan, 1990.

Alnasralla Mayar B., and Basel H. Nasralla. "Placebo Effects in Modern Medicine: Mechanisms, Clinical Evidence, Limitations, and Future Directions." *Cureus* Jan 2, 18, 1 (2026): e100612, doi: 10.7759/cureus.100612.

Ameijeiras Barros, Marta. "Rediscovering the Jacobean Cult in Medieval England: The Wall Paintings of St James the Great in Stoke Orchard." *Ad Limina* 6, no. 6 (2015): 221–49.

Amsler, Monika. "*Voces Magicae* and Imperial/Late-Antique World-Making. Part 1." *ASDIWAL. Revue genevoise d'anthropologie et d'histoire des religions* 16 (2021): 29–43.

Ankarloo, Bengt, and Stuart Clark. "Introduction." In *Witchcraft and Magic in Europe: 3. The Middle Ages*, ed. Karen L. Jolly, Catharina Raudvere, and Edward Peters, ix–xiv. The Athlone Press, 2002.

Anthony, Sean W. *Muhammad and the Empires of Faith: The Making of the Prophet of Islam*. University of California Press, 2020.

Ármann Jakobsson. *The Troll Inside You. Paranormal Activity in the Medieval North*. Punctum Books, 2017.

Arnovick, Leslie K. *Verbal Medicines. The Curative Power of Prayer and Invocation in Early English Charms*. Cambridge University Press, 2024.

Arthur, Ciaran. *"Charms," Liturgies, and Secret Rites in Early Medieval England*. Boydell&Brewer, 2018.

Austin, John L. *How to Do Things With Words*. Harvard University Press, 1962.

Bächtold-Stäubli, Hanns, and Eduard Hoffmann-Krayer, ed. *Handwörterbuch des deutschen Aberglaubens*. Vol. 8: *Silber–Vulkan*. De Gruyter, 1937.

Bader, Richard E. "Sator Arepo: Magik in der Volksmedizin." *Medizinhistorisches Journal* 22 (1987): 115–34.

Bagge, Sverre. *From Gang Leader to the Lord's Anointed. Kingship in Sverris saga and Hákonar saga Hákonarsonar*. Syddansk universitetsforlag, 1996.

Bakhouche, Béatrice, Frédéric Fauquier, and Brigitte Pérez-Jean. *Picatrix : Un traité de magie médiéval*. Brepols, 2003.

Banham, Debby. "Dun, Oxa and Pliny the Great Physician: Attribution and Authority in Old English Medical Texts." *Social History of Medicine* 24, no. 1 (2011): 57–73.

Banham, Debby. "England Joins the Medical Mainstream: New Texts in Eleventh-Century Manuscripts." In *Anglo-Saxon England and the Continent*, ed. Hans Sauer and Joanna Story, 341–51. Arizona Center for Medieval and Renaissance Studies, 2011.

Banham, Debby. "*Lectun* and *Orceard*: A Preliminary Survey of the Evidence for Horticulture in Anglo-Saxon England." In *The Anglo-Saxons: the World Through Their Eyes*, ed. Gale R.Owen-Crocker and Brian W. Schneider, 33–48. Archaeopress, 2014.

Banham, Debby. "The Old English Nine Herbs Charm." In *Medieval Christianity in Practice*, ed. Miri Rubin, 189–93. Princeton University Press, 2009.

Banham, Debby, and Christine Voth. "The Diagnosis and Treatment of Wounds in the Old English Medical Collections: Anglo-Saxon Surgery?," in *Wounds and Wound Repair in Medieval Culture*, ed. Kelly DeVries and Larissa Tracey, 153–74. Brill, 2015.

Barb, Alfons A. "The Survival of Magic Arts." In *The Conflict Between Paganism and Christianity in the Fourth Century*, ed. Arnaldo Momigliano, 100–25. Clarendon Press, 1963.

Barb, Alphonse A. "Bois du sang, Tantale." *Syria* 29, no. 3/4 (1952): 271–84.

Barrett-Lennard, R.J.S. *Healing after the New Testament: Some Approaches to Healing in the Second, Third, and Fourth Centuries*. University Press of America, 1994.

Bartlett, Robert. *Trial by Fire and Water. The Medieval Judicial Ordeal*. Clarendon Press, 1986.

Bauman, Richard, and Charles L. Briggs. "Poetics and Performance as Critical Perspectives on Language and Social Life." *Annual Review of Anthropology* 19 (1990): 59–89.

Bell, Catherine. *Ritual Theory, Ritual Practice*. Oxford University Press, 2009 [1992].

Benati, Chiara. "Painted Eyes, Magical Sieves and Carved Runes: Charms for Catching and Punishing Thieves in the Medieval and Early Modern Germanic Tradition." In *Magic and Magicians in the Middle Ages and the Early Modern Time. The Occult in Pre-modern Sciences, Medicine, Literature, Religion, and Astrology*, ed. Albrecht Classen, 149–218. De Gruyter, 2017.

Benedetti, Fabrizio, Alessandro Piedimonte, and Elisa Frisaldi. "How Do Placebos Work?" *European Journal of Psychotraumatology* 9, sup3 (2018): https://doi.org/10.1080/2.

Bhugra, Dinesh, and Antonio Ventriglio. "Do Cultures Influence Placebo Response?" *Acta Psychiatrica Scandinavica* 132, no. 4 (2015): 227–30.

Bickerman, Elias J. "Darius I, Pseudo-Smerdis, and the Magi." *Athenaeum* 58 (1978): 239–61.

Bidez, Joseph, and Franz Cumont. *Les mages hellénisés*. Les Belles Lettres, 1939.

Bjork, Robert, ed. and trans. *Old English Shorter Poems. Vol. 2. Wisdom and Lyric.* University Press for Dumbarton Oaks Medieval Library, 2014.

Black, Robert D. *Education and Society in Florentine Tuscany. Teachers, Pupils and Schools, c. 1250–1500*. Brill, 2007.

Black, Robert D. *Humanism and Education in Medieval and Renaissance Italy.* Cambridge University Press, 2001.

Blanco Cesteros, Miriam. "Written in Blood? Decoding Some Red Inks of the Greek Magical Papyri." In *Traces of Ink. Experiences of Philology and Replication*, ed. Lucia Raggetti, 33–56. Brill, 2021.

Bloch, Maurice. "Symbols, Song, Dance, and Features of Articulation: Is Religion an Extreme Form of Authority?" *Archives Européennes de Sociologie* 15 (1974): 55–81.

Bloom, Paul. "Religion Is Natural." *Developmental Science* 10, 1 (2007): 147–51.

Bohak, Gideon. "Jewish Magic in the Middle Ages." In *The Cambridge History of Magic and Witchcraft in the West: From Antiquity to the Present*, ed. David J. Collins, 268–99. Cambridge University Press, 2015.

Bohak, Gideon. "The Diffusion of the Greco-Egyptian Magical Tradition in Late Antiquity." In *Greco-Egyptian Interactions. Literature, Translation, and Culture, 500 BCE–300 CE*, ed. Ian Rutherford, 357–81. Oxford University Press, 2016.

Bonnerot, Olivier, Eleni Chronopoulou, and Ira Rabin. "Instrumental Analysis of the Inks from the Magical Papyrus P. Berol. Inv. 5026 (PGM ii / GEMF 30)." *Zeitschrift für Papyrologie und Epigraphik* 224 (2022): 267–73.

Bonser, Wilfrid. "The Significance of Colour in Ancient and Mediaeval Magic: With Some Modern Comparisons." *Man* 25 (1925): 194–98.

Borsje, Jacqueline, and Fergus Kelly. "'The Evil Eye' in Early Irish Literature and Law." *Celtica* 24 (2003): 1–39.

Borsje, Jacqueline. "Druids, Deer and 'Words of Power:' Coming to Terms with Evil in Medieval Ireland." In *Coping with Evil in Religion and Culture. Case Studies*, ed. Nelly Van Doorn-harder and Lourens Minnema, 25–49. Rodopi, 2008.

Borsje, Jacqueline. "Witchcraft and Magic." In *Medieval Ireland. An Encyclopedia*, ed. Seán Duffy, 518–20. Routledge, 2005.

Bortolani, Ljuba M. *Magical Hymns from Roman Egypt: A Study of Greek and Egyptian Traditions of Divinity*. Cambridge University Press, 2016.

Boudet, Jean-Patrice, and Jean-Charles Coulon. "La version arabe (*Ghāyat al-ḥakīm*) et la version latine du *Picatrix*. Points communs et divergences." *Cahiers de recherches médiévales et humanistes* 33 (2017): 67–101.

Bourdieu, Pierre. *Ce que parler veut dire: l'économie des échanges linguistiques*. Fayard, 1982.

Boustan, Ra'anan, and Joseph E. Sanzo. "Christian Magicians, Jewish Magic, and the Shared Magical Culture of Late Antiquity." *Harvard Theological Review* 110, no. 2 (2017): 217–40.

Boyer, Pascal. “Being Human. Religion: Bound to Believe?” *Nature* 455 (2008): 1038–39.

Bozóky, Edina. *Charmes et prières apotropaïques*. Brepols, 2003.

Bozóky, Edina. “Medieval Narrative Charms.” In *The power of Words. Studies on Charms and Charming in Europe*, ed. James Kapaló, Éva Pócs, and William Ryan, 101–15. Central European University Press, 2013.

Brashear, William, and Roy Kotansky. “A New Magical Formulary.” In *Magic and Ritual in the Ancient World*, ed. Paul Mirecki and Marvin Meyer, 3–24. Brill, 2002.

Breatnach, Caoimhín. “Book of Lismore.” In *Medieval Ireland. An Encyclopedia*, ed. Seán Duffy, 279–80. Routledge, 2005.

Bremmer, Jan N. “The Birth of the Term ‘Magic.’” *Zeitschrift für Papyrologie und Epigraphik* 126 (1999): 1–12.

Brim, Charles J. *Medicine in the Bible*. Froben Press, 1936.

Brouwer, René. “Stoic Sympathy.” In *Sympathy. A History*, ed. Eric Schliesser, 15–35. Oxford University Press, 2015.

Browe, Peter. “Die Eucharistie als Zaubermittel im Mittelalter.” *Archiv für Kulturgeschichte* 20 (1930): 134–54.

Browe, Peter. *De ordaliis*, 2 vols. Apud aedes Pont. Universitatis Gregorianae, 1932.

Browe, Peter. *Die eucharistischen Wunder des Mittelalters*. Müller und Seiffert, 1938.

Brown, Peter. *Religion and Society in the Age of Saint Augustine*. Faber&Faber, 1972.

Brown, Peter. “Society and the Supernatural: A Medieval Change.” *Daedalus* 104, no. 2 (1975): 133–51.

Brown, Peter. *The Cult of the Saints: Its Rise and Function in Latin Christianity*. The University of Chicago Press, 1981.

Brown, Rachel F. “‘Taste and See That the Lord is Sweet’ (Ps. 33:9): The Flavor of God in the Monastic West.” *The Journal of Religion* 86, no. 2 (2006): 169–204.

Browning, Robert. “Literacy in the Byzantine World.” *Byzantine and Modern Greek Studies* 4 (1978): 39–54 [repr.: Robert Browning, *History, Language and Literacy in the Byzantine World*. Variorum Reprints, 1989].

Brunet, Jacqueline, and Odile Redon, ed. *Tables Florentines. Écrire et manger avec Franco Sacchetti*. Stock, 1984.

Burnett, Charles. “Béziers as an Astronomical Center for Jews and Christians in the Mid-Twelfth Century.” *Aleph* 17, no. 2 (2017): 197–219.

Burnett, Charles. “East (and South) Asian Traditions in Astrology and Divination as Viewed from the West.” *Extrême-Orient Extrême-Occident* 35 (2013): 285–93.

Burnett, Charles. “Magic in the Court of Alfonso el Sabio: The Latin Translation of the *Ġāyat al-Ḥakīm*.” In *De Frédéric II à Rodolphe II. Astrologie, divination et magie dans les cours (XIIIe–XVIIe siècle)*, ed. Jean-Patrice Boudet, Martine Ostorero, and Agostino Paravicini Bagliani, 37–52. SISMEL – Edizioni del Galluzzo, 2017.

Burnett, Charles. “*Nīrānj*, a Category of Magic (almost) Forgotten in the Latin West.” In *Natura, scienze e società medievali: Studi in onore di Agostino Paravicini Bagliani*, ed. Claudio Leonardi and Francesco Santi, 37–66. SISMEL – Edizioni del Galluzzo, 2008.

Burnett, Charles. "Thābit ibn Qurra the Ḥarrānian on Taslimans and the Spirits of the Planets." *La Corónica*, 36, no. 1 (2007): 13–40.

Burnett, Charles. "The Theory and Practice of Powerful Words in Medieval Magical Texts." In *The Word in Medieval Logic, Theology and Psychology: Acts of the XIII International Colloquium of the Société Internationale pour l'Étude de la Philosophie Médiévale*, Kyoto, 27 September–1 October 2005, ed. Tetsuro Shimizu and Charles Burnett, 215–31. Brepols, 2009.

Burridge, Claire. *Carolingian Medical Knowledge and Practice, c. 775–990. New Approaches to Recipe Literature*. Brill, 2024.

Burridge, Claire. "Early Medieval Recipe Collections: Continuity, Change and the Carolingian Contest." In *Early Medieval Medicine in Context. Transmission, Translation and Transformation*, ed. Debby Banham, Claire Burridge, and Lea T. Olsan, 114–63. Boydell & Brewer, 2025.

Burridge, Claire. "Healing Body and Soul in Early Medieval Europe: Medical Remedies with Christian Elements." *Studies in Church History* 58 (2022): 46–67.

Bynum, Caroline Walker. *Holy Feast and Holy Fast: The Religious Significance of Food to Medieval Women*. University of California Press, 1990.

Bynum, Caroline Walker. "The Sacrality of Things: An Inquiry into Divine Materiality in the Christian Middle Ages." *Irish Theological Quarterly* 78, no. 1 (2012): 3–18.

Calhoun, Robert M. "The Gospel(-amulet) as God's Power for Salvation." *Early Christianity* 10 (2019): 21–55.

Callegari, Danielle. *Dante's Gluttons. Food and Society from the Convivio to the Comedy*. Amsterdam University Press, 2022.

Cameron, Malcolm L. "Anglo-Saxon Medicine and Magic." *Anglo-Saxon England* 17 (1988): 191–215.

Cameron, Malcolm L. "Bald's *Leechbook* and Cultural Interactions in Anglo-Saxon England." *Anglo-Saxon England* 19 (1990): 5–12.

Cameron, Malcolm L. "Bald's *Leechbook*: Its Sources and their Uses in its Compilation." *Anglo-Saxon England* 12 (1983): 153–82.

Cameron, Malcolm L. "The Sources of Medical Knowledge in Anglo-Saxon England." *Anglo-Saxon England* 11 (1982): 135–55.

Cameron, Malcolm L. *Anglo-Saxon Medicine*. Cambridge University Press, 1993.

Camporesi, Piero. *Il pane selvaggio*. Il Mulino, 1980.

Camporesi, Piero. *Il sugo della vita: simbolismo e magia del sangue*. Mondadori, 1988.

Camporesi, Piero. *La carne impassibile*. Il Saggiatore, 1983.

Camporesi, Piero. *La terra e la luna: alimentazione, folclore, società*. Il Saggiatore, 1989.

Caneva, Stefano G. "The Persea Tree from Alexander to Late Antiquity: A Contribution to the Cultural and Social History of Greco-Roman Egypt." *Ancient Society* 46 (2016): 39–66.

Cardini, Franco. "Il 'breve' (secoli XIV–XV): tipologia e funzione." *La Ricerca Folklorica* 5 (1982): 63–73.

Cardona, Giorgio R. "Gli amuleti scritti: un excursus comparativo." *La Ricerca Folklorica* 8 (1983): 91–97.

Cardona, Giorgio R. *Antropologia della scrittura*. Utet, 2009 [1981].

Carey, John. "The Three Rings Required of a Poet." *Ériu* 48 (1997): 41–58.

Cavallo, Guglielmo. *Lire a Byzance*. Les belles lettres, 2006.

Cavell, Megan. "Powerful Patens in the Anglo-Saxon Medical Tradition and Exeter Book Riddle 48." *Neophilologus* 101, no. 1 (2017): 129–38.

Christiansen, Thomas. "Manufacture of Black Ink in the Ancient Mediterranean." *The Bulletin of the American Society of Papyrologists* 54 (2017): 167–95.

Clanchy, Michael. "Did Mothers Teach their Children to Read?" In *Motherhood, Religion, and Society in Medieval Europe, 400–1400. Essays Presented to Henrietta Leyser*, ed. Conrad Leyser and Lesley Smith, 129–53. Routledge, 2011.

Clason, Christopher R. "Animal, Birds, and Fish in the Middle Ages." In *Handbook of Medieval Culture. Volume 1*, ed. Albrecht Classen, 18–54. De Gruyter, 2015.

Classen, Albrecht. "Magic in the Middle Ages and the Early Modern Age – Literature, Science, Religion, Philosophy, Music, and Art. An Introduction." In *Magic and Magicians in the Middle Ages and the Early Modern Time. The Occult in Pre-modern Sciences, Medicine, Literature, Religion, and Astrology*, ed. Albrecht Classen, 1–108. De Gruyter, 2017.

Clunies Ross, Margaret. "Self-Description in Egil's Poetry." In *Egil, the Viking Poet: New Approaches to 'Egils saga'*, ed. Laurence de Looze, Jón Karl Helgason, Russell Poole, and Torfi H. Tulinius, 75–91. University of Toronto Press, 2015.

Coley, David K. *The Wheel of Language. Representing Speech in Middle English Poetry, 1377–1422*. Syracuse University Press, 2012.

Coupland, John N., and John E. Hayes. "Physical Approaches to Masking Bitter Taste: Lessons from Food and Pharmaceuticals." *Pharmaceutical Research* 31 (2014): 2921–39.

Cunliffe, Barry. *Druids: A Very Short Introduction*. Oxford University Press, 2010.

Curtius, Ernst R. *European Literature and the Latin Middle Ages*, ed. Willard R. Trask, 7th ed. Princeton University Press, 1990.

d'Alverny, Marie-Thérèse. "Survivance de la magie antique." In *Antike und Orient im Mittelalter: Vorträge der Kölner Mediävistentagungen, 1956–1959*, ed. Paul Wilpert, Miscellanea Mediaevalia, Veröffentlichungen des Thomas-Instituts an der Universität Köln, vol. 1., 154–78. De Gruyter, 1962.

D'Aronco, Maria Amalia. "Anglo Saxon Plant Pharmacy and the Latin Medical Tradition." In *From Earth to Art: The Many Aspects of the Plant-World in Anglo-Saxon England. Proceedings of the First ASPNS Symposium*, University of Glasgow, 5–7 April 2000, ed. Carole P. Biggam, 133–51. Rodopi, 2003.

D'Aronco, Maria Amalia. "L'erbario anglosassone, un'ipotesi sulla data della traduzione." *Romanobarbarica* 13 (1994/95): 325–66.

D'Aronco, Maria Amalia. "The Transmission of Medical Knowledge in Anglo- Saxon England: The Voices of Manuscripts." In *Form and Content of Instruction in Anglo-Saxon England in the Light of Contemporary Manuscript Evidence: Papers Presented at the International Conference*, Udine, 6–8 April 2006, ed. Patrizia Lendinara, Loredana Lazzari, and Maria Amalia D'Aronco, 35–58. Brepols, 2007.

D'Avray, David L. "The Concept of Magic." In *The Routledge History of Medieval Magic*, ed. Sophie Page and Catherine Rider, 48–56. Routledge, 2019.

Darmstaedter, Ernst. "Die Sator-Arepo-Formel und ihre Erklarung." *Isis* 18 (1932): 322–29.

Davies, Owen. *Grimoires: A History of Magic Books*. Oxford University Press, 2009.

Davies, Owen. *Magic: A Very Short Introduction*. Oxford University Press, 2012.

De Bruyn, Theodore S. *Making Amulets Christian: Artefacts, Scribes, and Contexts*. Oxford University Press, 2017.

de Bruyn, Theodore S., and Jitse H.F. Dijkstra. "Greek Amulets and Formularies from Egypt Containing Christian Elements: A Checklist of Papyri, Parchments, Ostraka, and Tablets." *The Bulletin of the American Society of Papyrologists* 48 (2011): 163–216.

de Callataÿ, Godefroid. "Magia en al-Andalus: *Rasā'il Iḫwān al-Ṣafā', Rutbat al-Ḥakīm y Ġāyat al-Ḥakīm* (*Picatrix*)." *Al-Quanṭara* 34, no. 2 (2013): 297–344.

de Haro Sanchez, Magali, ed. *Écrire la magie dans l'antiquité : Actes du colloque international (Liège, 13–15 octobre 2011)*. Presses Universitaires de Liège, 2015.

De Looze, Laurence. "Poet, Poem and Poetic Process in Egils Saga *Skalla-Grímssonar*." *Arkiv för nordisk filologi* 104 (1989): 123–42.

de Martino, Ernesto. "Crisi della presenza e integrazione religiosa." *Aut-Aut* 31 (1956): 17–38.

de Martino, Ernesto. *Il mondo magico*. Boringhieri, 1948.

de Meyier, Karel A., and P.F.J. Obbema. *Codices Vossiani Latini*, Pars I: *Codices in folio*. Universitaire pers Leiden, 1973.

Delaurenti, Béatrice. "Acting through Words in the Middle Ages: Communication and Action in the Debates on the Power of Incantations." *Archives de sciences sociales des religions* 158, no. 2 (2012): 53–71.

Delaurenti, Béatrice. *La Puissance des mots : "Virtus verborum." Débats doctrinaux sur le pouvoir des incantations au Moyen Âge*. Les Éditions du Cerf, 2007.

Deonna, Waldemar. "Abra, Abraca: La croix-talisman de Lausanne." *Genava* 22 (1944): 116–37.

Dickie, Matthew W. *Magic and Magicians in the Greco-Roman World*. Routledge, 2001.

Dieleman, Jacco. "The Greco-Egyptian Magical Papyri." In *Guide to the Study of Ancient Magic*, ed. David Frankfurter, 283–321. Brill, 2019.

Dillmann, François-Xavier. "Runenmeister." *Reallexikon der Germanischen Altertumskunde*, vol. 25, 537–46. De Gruyter, 2003.

Dillmann, François-Xavier. "Seiður og shamanismi í Íslendingasögum." *Skáldskaparmál* 2 (1993): 20–33.

Dillmann, François-Xavier. *Les magiciens dans l'Islande ancienne. Études sur la représentation de la magie islandaise et de ses agents dans les sources littéraires norroises*. Kungl. Gustav Adolfs Akademien för svensk folkkultur, 2006.

Djerbi, M. "L'incantation mythique : noms et écriture." *Ethnologie française* 23, no. 1 (1993): 94–103.

Dooley, Ann. *Playing the Hero: Reading the Irish Saga Táin Bó Cúailnge*. University of Toronto Press, 2006.

Dornseiff, Franz. *Das Alphabet in Mystik und Magie*. Teubner, 1922.

Doyle, Conan. "*Dweorg* in Old English: Aspects of Disease Terminology." *Quaestio Insularis* 9 (2008): 99–117.

Dubuisson, Daniel. "Les talismans du roi Cormac et les trois functions." *Revue historique* 250, no. 508 (1973): 289–94.

Dugan, Frank M. "Seldom Just Food: Garlic in Magic and Medicine in European and Mediterranean Traditions." *Digest: A Journal of Foodways and Culture* 5, no. 1 (2016): 1–60.

Durkheim, Émile. *The Elementary Forms of Religious Life*, trans. J.W. Swain. Free Press, 1965 [1915].

Durocher, Onésyme. "De la bibliophagie." In *Miscellanies of the Philobiblon Society* 10, 195–210. Whittingham and Wilkins, 1866–67.

Eidelberg, Shlomo. "Trial by Ordeal in Medieval Jewish History: Laws, Customs and Attitudes." In *Proceedings of the American Academy for Jewish Research*, vols. 46/47, 105–20. Jubilee Volume (1928–29/1978–79), Part 1 (1979–1980).

Elsakkers, Marianne. "In Pain You Shall Bear Children (Gen 3:16): Medieval Prayers for a Safe Delivery." In *Women and Miracle Stories. A Multidisciplinary Exploration*, ed. Anne-Marie Korte, 179–209. Brill, 2004.

El-Tom, Abdullahi Osman. "Drinking the Koran: The Meaning of Koranic Verses in Berti Erasure." *Africa: Journal of the International African Institute* 55, 4 (1985): 414–31.

Enck Paul, and Sibylle Klosterhalfen. "Placebo Responses and Placebo Effects in Functional Gastrointestinal Disorders." *Front Psychiatry* Aug 25, 11, 797 (2020), doi: https://doi.org/10.3389/fpsyt.2020.00797.

Epstein, Wilhelm. *Die Medizin im Alten Testament*. Ferdinand Enke, 1901.

Eriksen, Stefka G. "'Liquid Knowledge' in Old Norse Literature and Culture." *Viator* 49, no. 2 (2018): 169–97.

Esposito, Mario. "Sur la 'Navigatio Sancti Brendani' et sur ses versions italiennes : I. – La *Navigatio*." *Romania* 64, no. 255 (1938): 328–46.

F. Kenney, James. “Religious Literature and Ecclesiastical Culture.” In Id., *The Sources for the Early History of Ireland: An Introduction and Guide. Volume 1: Ecclesiastical*, 622–744. Octagon, 1966.

Fahd, Toufic. “Siḥr.” In *Encyclopaedia of Islam, Second Edition*, ed. Peri Bearman, C. Edmund Bosworth, Edmund van Donzel et al.: http://dx.doi.org/10.1163/1573-3912_islam_SIM_7023.

Fanger, Claire, ed. *Conjuring Spirits: Texts and Traditions of Medieval Ritual Magic*. Pennsylvania State University Press, 1998.

Fanger, Claire. “For Magic: Against Method.” In *The Routledge History of Medieval Magic*, ed. Sophie Page and Catherine Rider, 26–36. Routledge, 2019.

Fanger, Claire. “Magic.” In *The Oxford Guide to the Historical Reception of Augustine*, ed. Karla Pollman and Willemien Otten, 3 vols., vol. 3, 860–5. Oxford University Press, 2013.

Faraone, Christopher A. *Ancient Greek Love Magic*. Harvard University Press, 1999.

Faraone, Christopher A. “Does Tantalus Drink the Blood, or Not? An Enigmatic Series of Inscribed Hematite Gemstones.” In *Antike Mythen Medien, Transformationen und Konstruktionen*, ed. Ueli Dill and Christine Walde, 203–28. De Gruyter, 2009.

Faraone, Christopher A. “Necromancy Goes Underground: The Disguise of Skull- and Corpse-Divination in the Paris Magical Papyri (*PGM* IV 1928–2144).” In *Mantikê. Studies in Ancient Divination*, ed. Sarah Iles Johnston and Peter T. Struck, 255–82. Brill, 2005.

Faraone, Christopher A. *The Transformation of Greek Amulets in Roman Imperial Times*. University of Pennsylvania Press, 2018.

Feinstein, Eve L. “The ‘Bitter Waters’ of Numbers 5:11–31.” *Vetus Testamentum* 62 (2012): 300–306.

Fernández Fernández, Laura. *Arte y ciencia en el* scriptorium *de Alfonso X el Sabio*. Universidad de Sevilla/Cátedra Alfonso X el Sabio, 2013.

Ferrari, Fulvio. *Le saghe nordiche. Eroi, vichinghi e poeti nella Scandinavia medievale*. Meltemi, 2022.

Fierro, Maribel. “Bāṭinism in al-Andalus: Maslama b. Qāsim al-Qurṭubī (d. 353/964), Author of the *Rutbat al- Ḥakīm* and the *Ghāyat al-Ḥakīm* (Picatrix).” *Studia Islamica* 84, no. 2 (1996): 87–112.

Filotas, Bernadette. *Pagan Survivals: Superstitions and Popular Cultures in Early Medieval Pastoral Literature*. Pontifical Institute of Mediaeval Studies, 2005.

Fiori, Roberto. “Ordalie e diritto romano.” *IURA. Rivista Internazionale di Diritto Romano e Antico* 65 (2017): 1–128.

Flint, Valerie I.J. “The Demonisation of Magic and Sorcery in Late Antiquity: Christian Redefinitions of Pagan Religions.” In *Magic and Witchcraft in Ancient Europe*, vol. II: *Ancient Greece and Rome*, ed. Bengt Ankarloo and Stuart Clark, 279–348. University of Pennsylvania Press, 1999.

Flint, Valerie I.J. "The Early Medieval *medicus*, the Saint – and the Enchanter." *Social History of Medicine* 2, no. 2 (1989): 127–45.

Flint, Valerie I.J. *The Rise of Magic in Early Medieval Europe*. Princeton University Press, 1991.

Flood, Finbarr Barry. "Bodies and Becoming. Mimesis, Mediation, and the Ingestion of the Sacred in Christianity and Islam." In *Sensational Religion. Sensory Cultures in Material Practice*, ed. Sally M. Promey, 459–93. Yale University Press, 2014.

Forcada, Miquel. "Astrology in al-Andalus during the Eleventh and Twelfth Centuries: Between Religion and Philosophy." In *From Masha'allah to Kepler: Theory and Practice in Medieval and Renaissance Astrology*, ed. Charles Burnett and Dorian Greenbaum, 149–76. Sophia Centre Press, 2015.

Forshaw, Peter J. "From Occult Ekphrasis to Magical Art Transforming Text into Talismanic Image in the Scriptorium of Alfonso X." In *Bild und Schrift auf "magischen" Artefakten*, ed. Sarah Kiyanrad, Christoffer Theis, and Laura Willer, 15–47. De Gruyter, 2018.

Foscati, Alessandra. "La scena del parto. Nascita del corpo e salvezza dell'anima tra religione, medicina e 'magia' nell'altomedioevo." In *La presenza dei bambini nelle religioni del Mediterraneo antico: la vita e la morte, i rituali e i culti tra archeologia, antropologia e storia delle religioni*, ed. Chiara Terranova, 311–37. Aracne, 2014.

Frankfurter, David. "Ancient Magic in a New Key: Refining an Exotic Discipline in the History of Religions." In *Guide to the Study of Ancient Magic*, ed. David Frankfurter, 3–20. Brill, 2019.

Frankfurter, David. "Ritual Expertise in Roman Egypt and the Problem of the Category 'Magician.'" In *Envisioning Magic: A Princeton Seminar and Symposium*, ed. Peter Schäfer and Hans G. Kippenberg, 115–35. Brill, 1997.

Frankfurter, David. "Syncretism and the Holy Man in Late Antique Egypt." *Journal of Early Christian Studies* 11 (2003): 339–85.

Frankfurter, David. "The Magic of Writing and the Writing of Magic. The Power of the Word in Egyptian and Greek Tradition." *Helios* 21 (1994): 189–221.

Frankfurter, David. "The Magic of Writing in Mediterranean Antiquity." In *Guide to the Study of Ancient Magic*, ed. David Frankfurter, 626–58. Brill, 2019.

Frankfurter, David. "The Theory and Practice of the Magical *Historiola* in Ritual Spell." In *Ancient Magic and Ritual Power*, ed. Marvin Meyer and Paul Mirecki, 455–76. Brill, 2001.

Frazer, James G. *The Golden Bough: A Study in Magic and Religion*, abridged ed. Macmillan, 1922.

Freeman, Charles. *Holy Bones, Holy Dust: How Relics Shaped the History of Medieval Europe*. Yale University Press, 2011.

French, Valerie. "Midwives and Maternity Care in the Greco-Roman World." *Helios* 13, no. 2 (1987): 69–84.

Frevel, Christian. "On Instant Scripture and Proximal Texts: Some Insights into the Sensual Materiality of Texts and their Ritual Roles in the Hebrew Bible and Beyond." *Postscripts: The Journal of Sacred Texts, Cultural Histories, and Contemporary Contexts* 8, no. 1–2 (2017): 57–79.

Friedmann, Daniel. *Diritto e morale nelle storie bibliche*, trans. Diana Zerilli. Giuffrè Editore, 2008.

Frymer-Kensky, Tikva. "The Strange Case of the Suspected Sotah (Numbers v 11–31)." *Vetus Testamentum* 34 (1984): 11–26.

Gaidoz, Henri. "Les gâteaux alphabétiques." *Mélanges Rénier. Recuil de travaux publiés par l'École Pratique des Hautes Études* 73 (1887): 1–8.

Galavaris, George. *Bread and the liturgy; the symbolism of early Christian and Byzantine bread stamps*. The University of Wisconsin Press, 1970.

Gamble, Joel L. "A Defense of the Carolingian 'Defense of Medicine:' Introduction, Translation, and Notes." *Traditio* 75 (2020): 87–125.

García Avilés, Alejandro. "La magie astrale comme art visuel au XIIIe siècle." In *Images et magie*. Picatrix *entre Orient et Occident*, ed. Jean-Patrice Boudet, Anna Caiozzo, and Nicolas Weill-Parot, 95–113. Champion, 2011.

Gardiner, Noah. "Books on Occult Sciences." In *Treasures of Knowledge: An Inventory of the Ottoman Palace Library (1502/3–1503/4). Volume I: Essays*, ed. Gülru Necipoğlu, Cemal Kafadar, and Cornell H. Fleischer, 735–65. Brill, 2019.

Garipzanov, Ildar. "Graphic Ciphers and the Early Medieval Practices of *Collectio* and Concealment." In *Crafting Knowledge in the Early Medieval Book: Practices of Collecting and Concealing in the Latin West*, ed. Sinéad O'Sullivan and Ciaran Arthur, 409–38. Brepols, 2023.

Garipzanov, Ildar. "Magical Charaktêres in the Carolingian World: A Ninth-Century Charm in MS Vat. lat. 5359 and Its Broader Cultural Context." *Speculum* 96, no. 2 (2021): 287–308.

Garner, Lori Ann. "Anglo-Saxon Charms in Performance." *Oral Tradition* 19, no. 1 (2004): 20–42.

Gaudemet, Jean. "Les ordalies au Moyen Âge: doctrine, législation et pratique canoniques." In Id., *La société ecclésiastique dans l'occident médiéval*, 99–135. Variorum Reprints, 1980.

Gautier, Alban. "Entre cuisine, médecine et magie : l'historien de l'alimentation face à quelques textes anglo-saxons." *Revue belge de Philologie et d'Histoire* 93, no. 2 (2015): 287–302.

Gayk, Shannon. "'Ete This Book:' Literary Consumption and Poetic Invention in Capgrave's Life of St. Katherine." In *Form and Reform. Reading across the Fifteenth Century*, ed. Shannon Gayk and Kathleen Tonry, 88–109. Ohio State University Press, 2011.

Geertz, Clifford. *The Interpretation of Cultures: Selected Essays by Clifford Geertz*. Basic Books, 2000 [1973].

Glotz, Gustav. *L'Ordalie dans la Grèce primitive : Étude de droit et de mythologie*. Fontemoing, 1904.

Goody, Jack, ed. *Literacy in traditional societies*. Cambridge University Press, 1968.

Goody, Jack. "Introduction." In *Literacy in traditional societies*, ed. Jack Goody, 1–26. Cambridge University Press, 1968.

Goody, Jack. "Restricted Literacy in Northern Ghana." In *Literacy in traditional societies*, ed. Jack Goody, 198–264. Cambridge University Press, 1968.

Gordon, Richard. "Charaktêres between Antiquity and Renaissance: Transmission and Re-invention." In *Les savoirs magiques et leur transmission de l'Antiquité à la Renaissance*, ed. Véronique Dasen and Jean-Michel Spieser, 253–300. SISMEL – Edizioni del Galluzzo, 2014.

Gordon, Richard. "*Charaktēres* between Antiquity and Renaissance: Transmission and Re-Invention." In *Les savoirs magiques et leur transmission de l'antiquité à la Renaissance*, ed. Véronique Dasen and Jean-Michel Spieser, 253–300. SISMEL – Edizioni del Galluzzo, 2014.

Gordon, Richard. "From Substance to Text: Three Materialities of 'Magic' in the Roman Imperial Period." In *The Materiality of Magic*, ed. Dietrich Boschung and Jan N. Bremmer, 133–76. Wilhlem Fink, 2015.

Graf, Fritz. "Prayer in Magic and Religious Ritual." In *Magika Hiera: Ancient Greek Magic and Religion*, ed. Christopher A. Faraone and Dirk Obbink, 188–97. Oxford University Press, 1991.

Graf, Fritz. "Magie et écriture : quelques réflexions." In *Écrire la magie dans l'antiquité : Actes du colloque international (Liège, 13–15 octobre 2011)*, 227–38. Presses Universitaires de Liège, 2015.

Grattan, J.H.G., and Charles Singer. *Anglo-Saxon Magic and Medicine*. Oxford University Press, 1952.

Green, Michael. "A Late Coptic Magical Text from the Collection of the Rijksmuseum van Oudheden, Leiden." *Oudheidkundige Mededelingen* 67 (1987): 29–43.

Green, Monica H. "The Development of the Trotula." *Revue d'Histoire des Textes* 26 (1996): 119–203.

Green, Monica H. *Women's Healthcare in the Medieval West*. Routledge, 2000.

Greenberg, Moshe. *Ezekiel 1–20: A New Translation with Introduction and Commentari*. Doubleday, 1983.

Greenwood, Susan. *The Anthropology of Magic*. Berg, 2009.

Greer, John M., and Christopher Warnock. *The Picatrix: Liber Rubeus Edition*. Adocentyn Press, 2011.

Grévin, Benoît, and Julien Véronèse. "Les 'caractères' magiques au Moyen Age (XIIe–XIVe siècle)." *Bibliothèque de l'École des Chartres* 162 (2004): 305–79.

Griffin, Carrie. "Historiography of Medieval Medicine." In *Handbook of Medieval Culture. Volume 1*, ed. Albrecht Classen, 651–66. De Gruyter, 2015.

Grig, Lucy. "Life and Death in Late Antiquity: Religious Rituals and Popular Culture." In *A Companion to Religion in Late Antiquity*, ed. Josef Lössl and Nicholas J. Baker-Brian, 455–73. Wiley Blackwell, 2018.

Grønlie, Siân. "Saint's Life and Saga Narrative." *Saga-Book* XXXVI (2012): 5–26.

Grosdidier de Matons, José. *Romanos le Mélode et les origines de la poésie religieuse à Byzance*. Beauchesne, 1977.

Haddad, Gérard. *Eating the Book: Dietary Rites and Paternal Function*, trans. David Jacobson. Agincourt Press, 2013.

HadžiMuhamedović, Safet. "My Grandmother Drank the Qur'an: Liquid Readings and Permeable Bodies in Bosnia." *CounterText* 7, no. 1 (2021): 73–89.

Hall, Alaric. *Elves in Anglo-Saxon England: Matters of Belief, Health, Gender and Identity*. Boydell Press, 2007.

Hallum, Bink. "New Light on Early Arabic Awfāq Literature." In *Islamicate Occult Sciences in Theory and Practice*, ed. Liana Saif, Francesca Leoni, Matthew Melvin-Koushki, and Farouk Yahya, 57–161. Brill, 2007.

Hamès, Constant, ed. *Coran et talismans. Textes et pratiques magiques en milieux musulman*. Karhthala, 2007.

Hartner, Willy. "Notes on Picatrix." *Isis* 56, no. 4 (1965): 438–51.

Hayden, Deborah. "From the 'King of the Waters' to Curative Manuscripts: Water and Medicine in Medieval Irish Textual Culture." In *The Elements in the Medieval World: Interdisciplinary Perspectives. Water*, ed. Marilina Cesario, Hugh Magennis, and Elisa Ramazzina, 75–98. Brill, 2024.

Hayden, Deborah. "Old English in the Irish Charms." *Speculum* 97, no. 2 (2022): 349–76.

Hayden, Deborah. "The Context and Obscure Language of Medical Charms in a Sixteenth-century Irish Remedy Book: Four Case Studies." In *Obscuritas in Medieval Irish and Welsh Literature*, ed. Chantal Kobel (forthcoming).

Healy, Margaret. "Wearing powerful words and objects: healing prosthetics." *Textual Practice* 30, no. 7 (2016): 1233–51.

Heide, Eldar. "Spinning *seiðr*." In *Old Norse religion in long-term perspectives. Origins, changes, and interactions*, ed. Anders Andrén, Kristina Jennbert, and Catharina Raudvere, 164–70. Nordic Academic Press, 200.

Heim, Richard. *Incantamenta magica Graeca latina*, Jahrbücher für classische Philologie, suppl. Bd XIX. Teubner, 1893.

Helleman, Wendy E. "Plotinus and Magic." *The International Journal of the Platonic Tradition* 4 (2010): 114–46.

Hen, Yitzhak. *Culture and Religion in Merovingian Gaul, A.D. 481–751*. Brill, 1995.

Hen, Yitzhak. "The Early Medieval West." In *The Cambridge History of Magic and Witchcraft in the West: From Antiquity to the Present*, ed. David J. Collins, 183–206. Cambridge University Press, 2015.

Henzen, Walter. "Der Rotulus von Mülinen. Codex 803 der Burgerbibliothek Bern." In *Geschichte, Deutung, Kritik: Literaturwissenschaftliche Beiträge dargebracht zum 65. Geburtstag Werner Kohlschmidts*, ed. Maria Bindschedler and Paul Zinsli, 13–27. Francke, 1969.

Hermann, Pernille. "Literacy." In *The Routledge Research Companion to the Medieval Icelandic Sagas*, ed. Ármann Jakobsson and Sverrir Jakobsson, 34–47. Routledge, 2017.

Hertz, Robert. "The Pre-Eminence of the Right Hand: A Study in Religious Polarity," trans. Rodney and Claudia Needham, *HAU: Journal of Ethnographic Theory* 3, no. 2 (2013): 335–57.

Heslop, Kate. "Hearing Voices: Uncanny Moments in the *Íslendingasögur*." *Gripla* XIX (2008): 93–122.

Heslop, Kate. "Talking Heads: The Mediality of Mímir." In *RE:writing. Medial Perspectives on Textual Culture in the Icelandic Middle Ages*, ed. Kate Heslop and Jürg Glauser, 63–84. Chronos, 2018.

Hindley, Katherine Storm. "Eating Words and Burning Them: The Power of Destruction in Medieval English Charm Texts." In *Zerstörung von Geschriebenem. Historische und transkulturelle Perspektiven*, ed. Carina Kühne-Wespi, Klaus Peter Oschema, and Joachim Friedrich Quack, 359–72. de Gruyter, 2019.

Hindley, Katherine Storm. "Text Over Time: The Written Word in English Charms Before 1350." *Incantatio* 7 (2018): 72–93.

Hindley, Katherine Storm. *Textual Magic. Charms and Written Amulets in Medieval England*. The University of Chicago Press, 2023.

Hofman, Rijcklof. "Durrow, Book of." In *The Encyclopaedia of Ireland*, ed. Brian Lalor, 330. Gill & Macmillan, 2003.

Hofmann, Anne. "Drinking Horns in Old Norse Culture: A Tradition Under Examination." *Analecta Archaeologica Ressoviensia* 10 (2015): 214–70.

Hollis, Stephanie. "Scientific and Medical Writings." In *A Companion to Anglo-Saxon Literature*, ed. Phillip Pulsiano and Elaine Treharne, 188–208, Blackwell, 2001.

Holman, J. Alan. *Pleistocene Amphibians and Reptiles in Britain and Europe*. Oxford University Press, 1998.

Holtsmark, Anne. "Kjærlighetsdiktning." In *Kulturhistorisk leksikon for nordisk middelalder*, ed. Johannes Brøndsted et al., 22 vols., VIII, 438–43. Rosenkilde og Bagger, 1956–78.

Honigmann, Ernest. "A Trial for Sorcery on August 22, A.D. 449." *Isis* 35, no. 4 (1944): 281–3.

Horden, Peregrine. "Sickness and Healing." In *The Cambridge History of Christianity 3: Early Medieval Christianities, c. 600–1100*, ed. Thomas F.X. Noble and Julia M.H. Smith, 416–32. Cambridge University Press, 2008.

Horden, Peregrine. "What's Wrong with Early Medieval Medicine?" *Social History of Medicine* 24, no. 1 (2011): 5–25.

Hui, C. Harry, Sing-Hang Cheung, Jasmine Lam, Esther Yuet Ying Lau, Livia Yuliawati, and Shu Fai Cheung. "In Search of the Psychological Antecedents and Consequences of Christian Conversion: A Three-Year Prospective Study." *Psychology of Religion and Spirituality* 9, no. 2 (2017): 220–30.

Hunt, Tony. *Popular Medicine in Thirteenth-Century England. Introduction and Texts.* Boydell&Brewer, 1990.

Hussain, Mohd K., Mohammad Saquib, Tanveer Ahamad, Shahnaaz Khatoon, and Mohammad Faheem Khan. "Mediterranean Cypress 'Cupressus sempervirens:' A Review on Phytochemical and Pharmacological Properties." *Current Traditional Medicine* 5, no. 4 (2019): 278–97.

Idel, Moshe. "On Talismanic Language in Jewish Mysticism." *Diogenes* 43, no. 2 (1995): 23–41.

Jacoby, Adolf. "Der Ursprung des Judicium offae." *Archiv für Religionswissenschaft* 13 (1910): 526–66.

Jacquart, Danielle, and Agostino Paravicini Bagliani, ed. *La Scuola Medica Salernitana. Gli autori e i testi.* SISMEL – Edizioni del Galluzzo, 2007.

James, Edward. "A Sense of Wonder: Gregory of Tours, Medicine, and Science." In *The Culture of Christendom. Essays in Medieval History in Commemoration of Denis L.T. Bethell*, ed. Marc A. Meyer, 45–60. Hambledon Press, 1993.

Janowitz, Naomi. *Icons of Power: Ritual Practices in Late Antiquity.* The Pennsylvania State University Press, 2002.

Janowitz, Naomi. *Magic in the Roman World. Pagans, Jews and Christians.* Routledge, 2001.

Janowitz, Naomi. "Water, Word and Name: The Shifting Pragmatics of the Sotah/Suspected Adulteress Ritual." In *Literature or Liturgy? Early Christian Hymns and Prayers in their Literary and Liturgical Context in Antiquity*, ed. Clemens Leonhard and Hermut Löhr, 15–31. Mohr Siebeck, 2014.

Jesch, Judith. "Runes and Verse: The Medialities of Early Scandinavian Poetry." *European Journal of Scandinavian Studies* 47, no. 1 (2017): 181–202.

Jesch, Judith, and Christina Lee. "Healing runes." In *Viking Encounters*, ed. Anne Pedersen and Søren Sindbæk, 386–98. Aarhus University Press, 2020.

Jexlev, Thelma. *Lokalarkiver til 1559: Gejstlige arkiver*, Bd. I: *Ærkestiftet og Roskilde stift*, Bd. 2: *Odense stift, jyske stifter og Slesvig stift. Rigsarkivet.* Rigsarkivet, 1973–1977.

Johnson-Sheehan, Richard, and Paul Lynch. "Rhetoric of Myth, Magic, and Conversion: A Prolegomena to Ancient Irish Rhetoric." *Rhetoric Review* 26, no. 3 (2007): 233–52.

Johnsson, J.W.S. "Henrik Harpestraeng. A Danish Salernitan." *Isis* 4, no. 1 (1921): 13–16.

Jolly, Karen L. "Anglo-Saxon Charms in the Context of a Christian World View." *Journal of Medieval History* 11 (1985): 279–93.

Jolly, Karen L. "Magic, Miracle, and Popular Practice in the Early Medieval West: Anglo-Saxon England." In *Religion, Science and Magic in Concert and in Conflict*, ed. Jacob Neusner, Ernest S. Fredrichs, and Paul Virgil McCraken Flesher, 166–82. Oxford University Press, 1989.

Jolly, Karen L. "Medieval Magic: Definitions, Beliefs, Practices." In *Witchcraft and Magic in Europe: 3. The Middle Ages*, ed. Karen L. Jolly, Catharina Raudvere, and Edward Peters, 1–72. The Athlone Press, 2002.

Jolly, Karen L. "Tapping the Power of the Cross: Who and for Who?" In *The Place of the Cross in Anglo-Saxon England*, ed. Catherine E. Karkov, Sarah L. Keefer, and Karen L. Jolly, 58–79. The Boydell Press, 2006.

Jolly, Karen L. *Popular Religion in Late Saxon England: Elf Charms in Context*. University of North Carolina Press, 1996.

Jones, Peter Murray, and Lea T. Olsan. "Performative Rituals for Conception and Childbirth in England, 900–1500." *Bulletin of the History of Medicine* 89, no. 3 (2015): 406–33.

Jordan, David. "Phallus or Fleas at Berol inv. 17202.31?" *Zeitschrift für Papyrologie und Epigraphik* 141 (2002): 139–41.

Kahl, Oliver, and Zeina Matar. "A Treatise on the Amicable Numbers 220 and 284 Attributed to Abū Maʿshar al-Balkhī." *Journal of Semitic Studies* 35, no. 2 (1990): 233–43.

Kahlos, Maijastina. "*Artis heu magicis*: The Lable of Magic in Fourth-Century Conflicts and Disputes." In *Pagans and Christians in Late Antique Rome. Conflict, Competition, and Coexistence in the Fourth Century*, ed. Michele Renee Salzman, Marianne Sághy and Rita Lizzi Testa, 162–177. Cambridge University Press, 2016.

Kaiser, Walter C. *Toward Old Testament Ethics*. Zondervan, 1983.

Keefer, Sarah Larratt. "*Ut in omnibus honorificetur Deus*: The *corsnæd* Ordeal in Anglo-Saxon England." In *The Community, the Family and the Saint. Patterns of Power in Early Medieval Europe*, ed Joyce M. Hill and Mary Swan, 237–64. Brill, 1998.

Kelly, Fergus. *A Guide to Early Irish Law*. Dublin Institute for Advanced Studies, 1988.

Kenney, James F. *The sources for the early history of Ireland: an introduction and guide*. Columbia University Press, 1929.

Kerff, Franz. "Frühmittelalterliche pharmazeutische Rezepte aus dem Kloster Tegernsee." *Sudhoffs Archiv* 67, no. 1 (1983): 111–16.

Kertzer, David I. *Ritual, Politics, and Power*. Yale University Press, 1988.

Kesling, Emily. *Medical Texts in Anglo-Saxon Literary Culture*. D.S. Brewer, 2020.

Kieckhefer, Richard. *Forbidden Rites: A Necromancer's Manual of the Fifteenth Century*. Pennsylvania State University Press, 1998.

Kieckhefer, Richard. *Magic in the Middle Ages*. Cambridge University Press, 1989.

Kieckhefer, Richard. "The Specific Rationality of Medieval Magic." *The American Historical Review* 99, no. 3 (1994): 813–36.

Klaes, Falko. *Mittelalterliche Glossen und Texte aus Trier. Studien zur volkssprachigen Trierer Überlieferung von den Anfängen bis zum Ende des 11. Jahrhunderts im lateinischen Kontext.* Universitätsverlag Winter, 2017.

Klapisch-Zuber, Christiane. "Le chiavi fiorentine di Barbablu: l'apprendimento della lettura a Firenze nel XV secolo." *Quaderni Storici* 57 (1984): 765–92.

Klingbeil, Gerald A. "'Eating' and 'Drinking' in the Book of Revelation: A Study of New Testament Thought and Theology." *Journal of the Adventist Theological Society* 16, no. 1–2 (2005): 75–92.

Klingshirn, William E. "Magic and Divination in the Merovingian World." In *The Oxford Handbook of the Merovingian World*, ed. Bonnie Effros and Isabel Moreira, 968–87. Oxford University Press, 2020.

Koering, Jérémie. *Iconophages. A History of Ingesting Images*, trans. Nicholas Huckle. Zone Books, 2024.

Koering, Jérémie. *Les iconophages: Une histoire de l'ingestion des images*. Actes Sud Éditions, 2021.

Koester, Craig R. *Revelation: A New Translation with Introduction and Commentary*. Yale University Press, 2014.

Kornbluth, Genevra. "Amulets and Identity in the Merovingian World." In *The Oxford Handbook of the Merovingian World*, ed. Bonnie Effros and Isabel Moreira, 941–67. Oxford University Press, 2020.

Korpelainen, Helena, and Maria Pietiläinen. "Sorrel (*Rumex acetosa* L.): Not Only a Weed but a Promising Vegetable and Medicinal Plant." *The Botanical Review* 86 (2020): 234–46.

Kössinger, Norbert. *Schriftrollen. Untersuchungen zu deutschsprachigen und mittelniederländischen Rotuli*. Reichert Verlag, 2020.

Köstler, Rudolf. "Der Anteil des Christentums an der Ordalien." *Zeitschrift der Savigny-Stiftung für Rechtsgeschichte: Kanonistische Abteilung* 32, 2 (1912): 208–48.

Kotansky, Roy D. "Textual Amulets and Writing Traditions in the Ancient World." In *Guide to the Study of Ancient Magic*, ed. David Frankfurter, 507–54. Brill, 2019.

Krappe, Alexander H. "St. Patrick and the Snakes." *Traditio* 5 (1947): 323–30.

Krause, Wolfgang, and Herbert Jankuhn, *Die Runeninschriften im älteren Futhark*. Vandenhoeck and Ruprecht, 1966.

Kruschwitz, Peter. "Inhabiting a Lettered World: Exploring the Fringes of Roman Writing Habits." *Bulletin of the Institute of Classical Studies* 59, no. 1 (2016): 26–41.

Kruschwitz, Peter. "Writing on Trees: Restoring a Lost Facet of the Graeco-Roman Epigraphic Habit." *Zeitschrift für Papyrologie und Epigraphik* 173 (2010): 45–62.

Künzler, Sarah. *Flesh and Word. Reading Bodies in Old Norse-Icelandic and Early Irish Literature*. de Gruyter, 2016.

L'Irlanda e gli irlandesi nell'alto medioevo. Atti della LVII Settimana di Studio (Spoleto 16–21 2009). CISAM, 2010.

Lacau, Pierre. "Les statues 'guérisseuses' dans l'ancienne Egypte." *Académie des inscriptions et belles-lettres. Commission de la fondation Poit, Monuments et Mémoires* 25 (1921–22): 189–209.

Lalatta Costerbosa, Marina. "Per una storia critica della tortura." *Materiali per una storia della cultura giuridica* 1 (2011): 3–34.

Lambek, Michael. "Certain Knowledge, Contestable Authority: Power and Practice on the Islamic Periphery." *American Ethnologist*. 17, no. 1 (1990): 23–40.

Láng, Benedek. "Characters and Magic Signs in the *Picatrix* and Other Medieval Magic Texts." *Acta Classica Universitatis Scientiarum Debreceniensis* 47 (2011): 69–77.

Lea, Henry C. *The Ordeal*. University of Pennsylvania Press, 1973 [1866].

Leclercq, Jean. *The Love of Learning and the Desire for God. A Study of Monastic Culture*. Fordham University Press, 1974 [1961].

Leja, Meg. *Embodying the Soul: Medicine and Religion in Carolingian Europe*. University of Pennsylvania Press, 2022.

Leja, Meg. "The Sacred Art: Medicine in the Carolingian Renaissance." *Viator* 47, no. 2 (2016): 1–34.

Lemesle, Bruno, ed. *La preuve en justice: de l'Antiquité à nos jours*. Presses universitaires de Rennes, 2003.

Leone, Massimo. "Le Dieu mâché. Idéologies du sens religieux et mastication." *Lexia. Rivista di semiotica* 19–20 (2015): 247–64.

Lethbridge, Emily. "Manuscripts and Textual Culture." In *The Cambridge History of Old Norse-Icelandic Literature*, ed. Heather O'Donoghue and Eleanor Parker, 33–49. Cambridge University Press, 2024.

Lévi-Strauss, Claude. "The Effectiveness of Symbols." In *Structural Anthropology 1*, ed. Claude Lévi-Strauss, 186–205. Penguin, 1949.

Looijenga, Tineke. *Texts & Contexts of the Oldest Runic Inscriptions*. Brill, 2003.

Lumby, Joseph Rawson. *Greek Learning in the Western Church during the Seventh and Eighth Centuries, A.D.* Cambridge, 1878.

MacLeod, Mindy, and Bernard Mees. *Runic Amulets and Magic Objects*. The Boydell Press, 2006.

Magennis, Hugh. *The Cambridge Introduction to Anglo-Saxon Literature*. Cambridge University Press, 2011.

Malinowski, Bronisław. *Coral Gardens and Their Magic*, 2 vols. Indiana University Press, 1935.

Malinowski, Bronisław. "Magic, Science and Religion." In Id., *Magic, Science, and Religion, and Other Essays*, 17–92. The Free Press, 1948.

Maraschi, Andrea. "Anthropophagy and Graphophagy in Medieval Scandinavia. Magic, Boundaries, and New Methodological Approaches to Food History." In *Entangled Food Histories. Methods and Sources for Exploring Foodways across Millennia*, ed.

Giacomo Casucci, Sofia Miola, Pietro Repishti and Sara Zanotta, 101–32. Edizioni dell'Orso, 2025.

Maraschi, Andrea. "Eaten Hearts and Supernatural Knowledge in *Eiríks saga rauða.*" *Scandia: Journal of Medieval Norse Studies* 1 (2018): 25–47.

Maraschi, Andrea. "Episodes of Cannibalism between Christians and Muslims from the Eleventh to the Thirteenth Centuries. Cases of Dehumanization and Hyper-Humanization." *Food, Culture & Society* (2024): https://doi.org/10.1080/15528014.2023.2300100.

Maraschi, Andrea. "I miracoli alimentari di San Colombano: l'originalità, la tradizione e la simbologia." *Studi Medievali* 52 (2011): 517–76.

Maraschi, Andrea. "Mangiare preghiere, bere incantesimi. Casi di grafofagia religiosa e magica nell'alto Medioevo." In *Medioevo misterioso*, ed. Paola Galetti, 99–115. Edizioni Scritture, 2024.

Maraschi, Andrea. "Nature, Supernature and the Human Body. Medicinal Remedies and Charms in Late Medieval Scandinavia." In *(Extra)Ordinary Bodies: Othered, Violated, and Devoured*, ed. Andrea Maraschi and Angelica A. Montanari, 70–80. Bookstones, 2023.

Maraschi, Andrea. "*Physis* e *Sympatheia*. Un corteo simpatetico femminile per invocare la pioggia nella Renania dell'anno 1000." In *"Con tuono, lampo o pioggia." Magia e stregoneria tempestarie fra antichità ed età moderna*, ed. Vincenzo Tedesco, 87–126. La Vela, 2023.

Maraschi, Andrea. Similia similibus curantur. *Cannibalismo, grafofagia e "magia" simpatetica nel Medioevo (500–1500)*. CISAM, 2020.

Maraschi, Andrea. "Sympathetic Graphophagy in Late Medieval Scandinavian Leechbooks and Collections of Charms." In *Civilizations of the Supernatural: Witchcraft, Ritual, and Religious Experience in Late Antique, Medieval, and Renaissance Traditions*, ed. Fabrizio Conti, 247–64. Trivent Publishing, 2020.

Maraschi, Andrea. "Sympathy for the Lord: The Host and Elements of Sympathetic Magic in Late Medieval Exempla." *Journal of Medieval Religious Cultures* 43, no. 2 (2017): 209–30.

Maraschi, Andrea. "The Impact of Christianization on Identity-Marking Foods in the Medieval North: Between Pagan Survivals, New Dietary Restrictions, and Magic Practice." *Food&History* 17, no. 2 (2020): 153–81.

Maraschi, Andrea. "Writing on Bread. Remarks on Cultural and Practical Boundaries Starting from a Fourteenth-Century Commonplace Book." In *Medieval Borders and the Environment*, ed. Elisa Ramazzina. Brill, forthcoming.

Maraschi, Andrea, and Francesca Tasca. "Aux limites de l'hérésie et de la magie. L'ordalie du pain et du fromage." *Food&History* 16, no. 1 (2018): 49–67.

Maraschi, Andrea, and Francesca Tasca. *Food, Heresies, and Magical Boundaries in the Middle Ages*. Amsterdam University Press, 2024.

Maréchal, Sadi. *Public Baths and Bathing Habits in Late Antiquity. A Study of the Evidence from Italy, North Africa and Palestine A.D. 287–700*. Brill, 2020.

Margo, Curtis E. "The Placebo Effect." *Survey of Ophthalmology* 44, no. 1 (1999): 31–44.

Markus, Robert A. "Signs, communication and communities in Augustine's *De doctrina christiana*." In De doctrina Christiana: *A Classic of Western Culture*, ed. Duane W.H. Arnold and Pamela Bright, 97–108. University of Notre Dame Press, 1995.

Marquès-Rivière, Jean. *Amulettes, talismans et pentacles dans les traditions orientales et occidentales*. Payot, 1972.

Martínez, Jesús Montoya. "El culto a la Eucaristía y sus derivaciones mágicas en el siglo XIII." *La corónica: A Journal of Medieval Hispanic Languages, Literatures, and Cultures* 36, no. 1 (2007): 189–96.

Matton, Sylvain. "An Irradiation of Latin Grammarians, or The *De radiis* Is Not by al-Kindī." *Magic, Ritual, and Witchcraft* 17, no. 3 (2022): 437–55.

Mauss, Marcel. *A General Theory of Magic*, trans. Robert Brain. W.W. Norton, 1972[1902].

McAuley, Finbarr. "Canon Law and the End of the Ordeal." *Oxford Journal of Legal Studies* 26, 3 (2006): 473–513.

McCartney, Eugene S. "Verbal Homeopathy and the Etymological Story." *The American Journal of Philology* 48, no. 4 (1927): 326–30.

McCutcheon, Russel T. *The insider/outsider problem in the Study of Religion*. Cassel, 1999.

McKinnell, John, Rudolf Simek, and Klaus Düwel. *Runes, Magic and Religion. A Sourcebook*. Fassbaender, 2004.

McNally, Robert E. "Medieval Exegesis." *Theological Studies* 22 (1961): 445–54.

McVaugh, Michael. "Incantationes in Late Medieval Surgery." In *Ratio et Superstitio: Essays in Honor of Graziella Federici Vescovini*, ed. Giancarlo Marchetti, Orsolo Rignani, and Valeria Sorge, 319–45. Fédération Internationale des Instituts d'Études Médiévales, 2003.

Meaney, Audrey L. "Extra-medical Elements in Anglo-Saxon Medicine." *Social History of Medicine* 24, no. 1 (2011): 41–56.

Meaney, Audrey L. "The Practice of Medicine about the Year 1000." *Social History of Medicine* 13, no. 2 (2000): 221–37.

Meaney, Audrey L. "Variant Versions of Old English Medical Remedies and the Compilation of Bald's Leechbook." *Anglo-Saxon England* 13 (1984): 235–68.

Meehan, Bernard. *The Book of Durrow: a medieval masterpiece at Trinity College Dublin*. Town House and Country House, 1996.

Meens, Rob. "Magic and the Early Medieval World View." In *The Community, the Family, and the Saint. Patterns of Power in Early Medieval Europe*, ed. Joyce M. Hill and Mary Swan, 285–95. Brepols, 1998.

Mees, Bernard. *The English Language Before England. An Epigraphic Account*. Routledge, 2023.

Mees, Bernard. "The Noleby inscription and Germanic *rehana." *Arkiv för nordisk filologi* 133 (2018): 5–28.

Mennella, Julie A., Alan C. Spector, Danielle R. Reed, and Susan E. Coldwell. "The Bad Taste of Medicines: Overview of Basic Research on Bitter Taste." *Clinical Therapeutics* 35, no. 8 (2013): 1225–46.

Metzger, Nadine. "Kynanthropy: Canine Madness in Byzantine Late Antiquity." *History of Psychiatry* 26, no. 3 (2015): 318–31.

Meyer, Marvin, and Paul Mirecki. "Introduction." In *Ancient Magic and Ritual Power*, ed. Marvin Meyer and Paul Mirecki, 1–11. Brill, 2001.

Meyer, Marvin, and Richard Smith. "Introduction." In *Ancient Christian Magic. Coptic Texts of Ritual Power*, ed. Marvin Meyer and Richard Smith, 1–9. HarperCollins, 1994.

Meylan, Nicolas. *Magic and Kingship in Medieval Iceland. The Construction of a Discourse of Political Resistance*. Brepols, 2014.

Meylan, Nicolas. "The Magical Power of Poetry." *Saga-Book* XXXVII (2013): 43–60.

Mineka, Susan, and Arne Öhman. "Phobias and Preparedness: The Selective, Automatic, and Encapsulated Nature of Fear." *Biological Psychiatry* 52, no. 10 (2002): 927–37.

Mitchell, Stephen A. "Anaphrodisiac Charms in the Nordic Middle Ages: Impotence, Infertility, and Magic." *Norveg* 38 (1998): 19–42.

Mitchell, Stephen A. "Magic and Religion." In *The Pre-Christian Religions of the North. History and Structures, Volume I: Basic Premises and Consideration of Sources*, ed. Jens Peter Schjødt, John Lindow, and Anders Andrén, 643–70. Brepols, 2020.

Mitchell, Stephen A. "Magic as Acquired Art and the Ethnographic Value of the Sagas." In *Old Norse Myths, Literature and Society*, ed. Margaret Clunies-Ross, 132–52. University Press of Southern Denmark, 2003.

Mitchell, Stephen A. "Scandinavia." In *The Routledge History of Medieval Magic*, ed. Sophie Page and Catherine Rider, 136–49. Routledge, 2019.

Mitchell, Stephen A. "*Skírnismál* and Nordic Charm Magic." In *Reflections on Old Norse Myths*, ed. Pernille Hermann, Jens Peter Schjødt, and Rasmus Tranum Kristensen, 75–94. Brepols, 2007.

Mitchell, Stephen A. *Witchcraft and Magic in the Nordic Middle Ages*. University of Pennsylvania Press, 2011.

Mohr, Christine, Lise Lesaffre, and Gustav Kuhn. "Magical Potential: Why Magic Performances Should be Used to Explore the Psychological Factors Contributing to Human Belief Formation." *Integrative Psychological and Behavioral Science* 53 (2019): 126–37.

Montanari, Massimo. *Il cibo come cultura*. Laterza, 2006.

Montesano, Marina. *Ars Magica. Una storia in 20 oggetti*. Carocci, 2025.

Montesano, Marina. *«Supra acqua et supra vento». "Superstizioni,"* maleficia e incantamenta *nei predicatori francescani osservanti (Italia, sec. XV)*. Istituto Storico Italiano per il Medio Evo, 1999.

Morenghi, Erminio. "Trotula de' Ruggiero e la Scuola medica salernitana. Una pioniera della medicina per le donne fatta da una donna." *Italies* 27 (2023): 93–106.

Morrison, Tessa. "The Art of Early Medieval Number Symbolism." *Journal of the Australian Early Medieval Association* 2 (2006): 169–81.

Motz, Lotte. "Of Elves and Dwarfs." *Arv: Journal of Scandinavian Folklore* 29–30 (1973–74): 93–127.

Napier, Arthur S. "Altenglische Miscellen." *Archiv für das Studium der neueren Sprachen und Literaturen* 83, no. 4 (1890): 323–27.

Nic Dhonnchadha, Aoibheann. "Medical Writing in Irish." *Irish Journal of Medical Science* 169 (2000): 217–20.

Nicolotti, Andrea. "A Cure for Rabies or a Remedy for Concupiscence? A Baptism of the Elchasaites." *Journal of Early Christian Studies* 16, no. 4 (2008): 513–34.

Nieber, Hanna. "'They All Just Want to Get Healthy!' Drinking the Qur'an between Forming Religious and Medical Subjectivities in Zanzibar." *Journal of Material Culture* 22, no. 4 (2017): 453–75.

Niles, John D. "Trial by Ordeal in Anglo-Saxon England: What's the Problem with Barley?" In *Early Medieval Studies in Memory of Patrick Wormald*, ed. Stephen Baxter, Catherine Karkov, Janet L. Nelson, and David Pelteret, 369–82. Routledge, 2009.

Nutton, Vivian. "Early Medieval Medicine and Natural Science." In *The Cambridge History of Science 2: Medieval Science*, ed. David C. Lindberg and Michael H. Shank, 323–40. Cambridge University Press, 2013.

Nutton, Vivian. "From Medical Certainty to Medical Amulets: Three Aspects of Ancient Therapeutics." *Essays in the History of Therapeutics*, ed. Carolyne Walker Bynum and Vivian Nutton, 13–22. Brill, 1991.

Nutton, Vivian. "Medicine in Late Antiquity and the Early Middle Ages." In *The Western Medical Tradition: 800 BC to AD 1800*, ed. Laurence I. Conrad, Michael Neve, Vivian Nutton, Roy Porter, and Andrew Wear, vol. 1, 71–87. Cambridge University Press, 1995.

Ó Concheanainn, Tomás. "The Scribe of the Leabhar Breac." *Ériu* 24 (1973): 64–79.

Ó Corráin, Donnchadh, ed. Clavis Litterarum Hibernensium: *Medieval Irish Books & Texts (c. 400–c. 1600)*. Brepols, 2017.

Ó Cuív, Brian. "Observations on the Book of Lismore." *Proceedings of the Royal Irish Academy. Section C: Archaeology, Celtic Studies, History, Linguistics, Literature* 83C (1983): 269–92.

Ó Riain-Raedel, Dagmar. "The Other Paradise: Perceptions of Ireland in the Middle Ages." In *Between the Islands and the Continent: Papers on Hiberno-Scandinavian-Continental Relations in the Early Middle Ages*, ed. Rudolf Simek and Asya Ivanova, 167–92. Fassbaender, 2013.

O'Donnell, Daniel P. *Cædmon's Hymn: A multimedia study, archive and edition.* D.S. Brewer, SEENET, and The Medieval Academy, 2005.

O'Reilly, Jennifer. *History, Hagiography and Biblical Exegesis. Essays on Bede, Adomnán and Thomas Becket.* Routledge, 2019.

Odell, Margaret S. "You Are What You Eat: Ezekiel and the Scroll." *Journal of Biblical Literature* 117, no. 2 (1998): 229–48.

Ogden, Charles Kay, and Ivor A. Richards. *The Meaning of Meaning.* Kegan Paul, 1923.

Olsan, Lea T. "Charms and Prayers in Medieval Medical Theory and Practice." *Social History of Medicine* 16, no. 3 (2003): 343–66.

Olsan, Lea T. "Charms in Late Antiquity and Early Medieval Medicine: Transmission and Transformation." In *Early Medieval Medicine in Context. Transmission, Translation and Transformation*, ed. Debby Banham, Claire Burridge, and Lea T. Olsan, 166–204. Boydell&Brewer, 2025.

Olsan, Lea T. "Latin Charms of Medieval England: Verbal Healing in a Christian Oral Tradition." *Oral Tradition* 7, no. 1 (1992): 116–42.

Olsan, Lea T. "Writing on the Hand in Ink: A Late Medieval Innovation in Fever Charms in England." *Incantatio* 7 (2018): 9–45.

Ong, Walter J. *Interfaces of the Word.* Cornell University Press, 1977.

Ong, Walter J. *Orality and Literacy: The Technologizing of the Word.* Methuen, 1982.

Önnerfors, Alf. "Magische Formel nim Dienste römischer Medizin." In *Aufstieg und niedergang der römischen Welt*, ed. Wolfgang Haase and Hildegard Temporini, II, 37.1, 157–224. De Gruyter, 1993.

Orchard, Andy. "The Word Made Flesh: Christianity and Oral Culture in Anglo-Saxon Verse." *Oral Tradition* 24, no. 2 (2009): 293–318.

Otto, Bernd-Christian. "A Discourse Historical Approach Towards Medieval Learned Magic." In *The Routledge History of Medieval Magic*, ed. Sophie Page and Catherine Rider, 37–47. Routledge, 2019.

Otto, Bernd-Christian. "Historicising 'Western Learned Magic:' Preliminary Remarks." *Aries* 16, no. 2 (2016): 161–240.

Otto, Bernd-Christian. *Magie. Rezeptions- und diskursgeschichtliche Analysen von der Antike bis zur Neuzeit.* De Gruyter, 2011.

Paden, William D., and Frances Freeman Paden. "Swollen Woman, Shifting Canon: A Midwife's Charm and the Birth of Secular Romance Lyric." *Publications of the Modern Language Association* 125, no. 2 (2010): 306–21.

Page, Raymond I. *Runes and Runic Inscriptions: Collected Essays On Anglo-Saxon and Viking Runes.* The Boydell Press, 1995.

Page, Sophie. "Medieval Magic." In *The Oxford History of Witchcraft and Magic*, ed. Owen Davies, 29–61. Oxford University Press, 2023.

Pagani, Roberto. "The Mediterranean Origin of the *Galdrastafir*. Tracing the Transmission of the Learned European Magical Tradition into Icelandic Popular Lore." *Gripla* 36 (2025): 241–69.

Palmer, James T. "Merovingian Medicine Between Practical Art and Philosophy." *Traditio* 89 (2023): 17–45.

Palmer, James T. *Merovingian Worlds*. Cambridge University Press, 2025.

Palmieri, Matteo. *Vita civile*, ed. Gino Belloni. Sansoni, 1982.

Papaioannou, Stratis. "Authors." In *The Oxford Handbook of Byzantine Literature*, 483–524. Oxford University Press, 2021.

Park, Katharine. "Medicine and Society in Medieval Europe, 500–1500." In *Medicine in Society: Historical Essays*, ed. Andrew Wear, 59–90. Cambridge University Press, 1992.

Parnell, Suzanne Sheldon, and Lea T. Olsan. "The Index of Charms: Purpose, Design, and Implementation." *Literary and Linguistic Computing* 6, no. 1 (1991): 59–63.

Patzuk-Russell, Ryder. *The Development of Education in Medieval Iceland*. De Gruyter, 2021.

Perreaut, Gaïa. "'Þú Eigir Illa Móður:' Of Cunning Kerlings and *fjǫlkynngi* – Disrupting Social Cohesion Through Magic." In *Performing Magic in the Pre-Modern North. Practice and Transgressions*, ed. Jennifer Hemphill, Ségdae Richardson-Read, and Solveig Marie Wang, 215–38. Palgrave Macmillan, 2024.

Pingree, David. "Some of the Sources of the Ghāyat al-hakīm." *Journal of the Warburg and Courtauld Institutes* 43 (1980): 1–15.

Piras, Andrea. *Verba lucis. Scrittura, immagine e libro nel manicheismo*. Mimesis, 2012.

Poole, Russell. "Charms and Incantations." In *Handbook of Medieval Culture. Volume 1*, ed. Albrecht Classen, 1700–1705. De Gruyter, 2015.

Poulin, Joseph-Claude. "Entre la magie et la religion. Recherches sur les utilisations marginales de l'écrit dans la culture populaire du haut Moyen Age." In *La culture populaire au Moyen Âge*, ed. Pierre Boglioni, 123–43. Les Éditions Univers, 1979.

Powell, Roger. "The Book of Kells, the Book of Durrow. Comments on the vellum, the make-up and other aspects." *Scriptorium* 10, no. 1 (1956): 3–21.

Preuss, Julius. *Biblical and Talmudic Medicine*, trans. Fred Rosner. Jason Aronson, 1993.

Price, Neil. *The Viking Way. Magic and Mind in Late Iron Age Scandinavia*. Oxbow, 2019.

Price, Neil. *The Viking Way: Religion and War in Late Iron Age Scandinavia*. Uppsala universitet, Department of Archaeology and Ancient History, 2002.

Pringle, Reginald D. "Traditions Relating to St James the Great in the Accounts of Medieval Latin Pilgrims to the Holy Land." In *Translating the Relics of St James: From Jerusalem to Compostela*, ed. Antón M. Pazos, 123–39. Routledge, 2017.

Pritchard, Melissa. "On Bibliomancy, Anthropodermic Bibliopegy, and The Eating Papers; or, Proust's Porridge." *Speaking Volumes* 63 (2014): 26–35.

Pucci Donati, Francesca. *Dieta, salute, calendari: dal regime stagionale antico ai* regimina mensium *medievali: origine di un genere nella letteratura medica occidentale*. CISAM, 2007.

Quinn, Judy. "From Orality to Literacy in Medieval Iceland." In *Old Icelandic Literature and Society*, ed. Margaret Clunies Ross, 30–60. Cambridge University Press, 2000.

Quinn, Judy. "Liquid Knowledge: Traditional Conceptualisation of Learning in Eddic Poetry." In *Along the Oral-Written Continuum: Types of Texts, Relations and their Implications*, ed. Slavika Rankovič, Leidulf Melve, and Else Mundal, 183–226. Brepols, 2010.

Quinn, Judy. "Verse Form and Voice in Eddic Pomes: The Discourses of *Fáfnismál*." *Arkiv för nordisk filologi* 107 (1992): 100–30.

Rabin, Ira. "Material Studies of Historic Inks: Transition from Carbon to Iron-Gall Inks." in *Traces of Ink. Experiences of Philology and Replication*, ed. Lucia Raggetti, 70–8. Brill, 2021.

Rampton, Martha. *Trafficking with Demons. Magic, Ritual, and Gender from Late Antiquity to 1000*. Cornell University Press, 2021.

Rappaport, Roy A. *Ritual and Religion in the Making of Humanity*. Cambridge University Press, 1999.

Rashed, Roshdi, and Christian Houzel. "Théorie des nombres amiables." In *Thābit ibn Qurra. Science and Philosophy in Ninth-Century Baghdad*, ed. Roshdi Rashed, 77–151. De Gruyter, 2009.

Raudvere, Catharina. "The Power of the Spoken Word as Literary Motif and Ritual Practice in Old Norse Literature." *Viking and Medieval Scandinavia* 1 (2005): 179–202.

Raudvere, Catharina. "*Trolldómr* in Early Medieval Scandinavia." In *Witchcraft and Magic in Europe. Vol. 3. The Middle Ages*, ed. Karen L. Jolly, Catharina Raudvere, and Edward Peters, 73–171. The Athlone Press, 2002.

Rausing, Gad. "On the origin of the runes." *Fornvännen* 87 (1992): 200–205.

Reider, Paula M. "Pregnancy and Childbirth: Christian Women." In *Women and Gender in Medieval Europe: An Encyclopedia*, ed. Margaret Schaus, 666–68. Routledge, 2006.

Remus, Harold. "'Magic,' Method, Madness." *Method & Theory in the Study of Religion* 11, no. 3 (1999): 258–98.

Reynolds, Leighton D. *Texts and Transmissions: A Survey of Latin Classics*. Clarendon Press, 1983.

Reynolds, Suzanne. *Medieval Reading: Grammar, Rhetoric and the Classical Text*. Cambridge University Press, 1996.

Richter, Michael. "Medieval Ireland and Iceland – Worlds Apart?" In *Saluting Aron Gurevich. Essays in History, Literature and Other Related Subjects*, ed. Yelena Mazour-Matusevich and Alexandra Korros, 155–66. Brill, 2010.

Ricks, Stephen D. "The Magician as Outsider in the Hebrew Bible and the New Testament." In *Ancient Magic and Ritual Power*, ed. Marvin Meyer and Paul Mirecki, 131–43. Brill, 2001.

Riddle, John M. "Women's Medicines in Ancient Jewish Sources: Fertility Enhancers and Inhibiters." In *Disease in Babylonia*, ed. Irving L. Finkel and Markham J. Geller, 200–214. Brill, 2007.

Ritari, Katja. "From Pagan to Christian in the 7th century Irish Hagiography." *Studia Celtica Fennica* 1 (2004): 14–23.

Ritner, Robert K. "Horus on the Crocodiles: A Juncture of Religion and Magic in Late Dynastic Egypt." In *Religion and Philosophy in Ancient Egypt*, ed. William K. Simpson, 103–16. Yale University Press, 1989.

Ritner, Robert K. *The Mechanics of Ancient Egyptian Magical Practice*. The Oriental Institute of the University of Chicago, 1993.

Ritter, Hellmut, and Martin Plessner. *"Picatrix:" Das Ziel des Weisen von Mağrīṭī*. Warburg Institute, 1962.

Ronconi, Filippo, and Stratis Papaioannou. "Book Culture." In *The Oxford Handbook of Byzantine Literature*, 44–75. Oxford University Press, 2021.

Roper, Jonathan. *Charms and Charming in Europe*. Springer, 2004.

Rosengren, Karl S., and Jason A. French. "Magical Thinking." In *The Oxford Handbook of the Development of Imagination*, ed. Marjorie Taylor, 42–60. Oxford University Press, 2013.

Rosenmeyer, Patricia A. *Ancient Epistolary Fictions: The Letter in Greek Literature*. Cambridge University Press, 2001.

Rosner, Fred. *Medicine in the Bible and the Talmud*. Yeshiva University Press, 1995.

Ross, Anne. "Ritual and the Druids." In *The Celtic World*, ed. Miranda J. Green, 423–44. Routledge, 1995.

Rozin, Paul, Linda Millman, and Carl Nemeroff. "Operation of the Laws of Sympathetic Magic in Disgust and Other Domains." *Journal of Personality and Social Psychology* 50, no. 4 (1986): 703–12.

Rozin, Paul, Maureen Markwith, and Bonnie Ross. "The Sympathetic Magical Law of Similarity, Nominal Realism, and Neglect of Negatives in Response to Negative Labels." *Psychological Science* 1, no. 6 (1990): 383–84.

Russell, Jeffrey B. *Witchcraft in the Middle Ages*. Cornell University Press, 1972.

Saif, Liana. *The Arabic Influences on Early Modern Occult Philosophy*. Palgrave MacMillan, 2015.

Savage-Smith, Emilie. "Medicine in Medieval Islam." In *The Cambridge History of Science*, ed. David C. Liindberg and Michael H. Shank, 139–67. Cambridge University Press, 2013.

Sävborg, Daniel. "Painful Love and Desire in Skírnismál: Origins and Contexts." In *The Wild Hunt for Numinous Knowledge: Perspectives on and from the Study of Pre-Christian Nordic Religion in Honour of Jens Peter Schjødt*, ed. Karen Bek-Pedersen, Sophie Bønding, Luke John Murphy, Simon Nygaard, and Morten Warmind, *Religionsvidenskabeligt Tidsskrift* 74 (2022): 490–512.

Sax, William, Johannes Quack, and Jan Weinhold, ed. *The Problem of Ritual Efficacy*. Oxford University Press, 2010.

Sayers, William. "Poetry and Social Agency in *Egils saga Skalla-Grímssonar*." *Scripta Islandica* 45 (1995): 29–62.

Schäfer, Peter. "Jewish Magic Literature in Late Antiquity and the Early Middle Ages." *Journal of Jewish Studies* 41 (1990): 75–91.

Schliesser, Eric. "Introduction: On Sympathy." In *Sympathy. A History*, ed. Eric Schliesser, 3–14. Oxford University Press, 2015.

Schmidt, Brian B. "Canaanite Magic vs. Israelite Religion: Deuteronomy 18 and the Taxonomy of Taboo." In *Magic and Ritual in the Ancient World*, ed. Paul Mirecki and Marvin Meyer, 242–59. Brill, 2002.

Schmidt, Paul G. "Il libro come medicina: la biblioterapia." Trans. Iolanda Ventura. In *Terapie e guarigioni. Convegno internazionale (Ariano Irpino, 5–7 Ottobre 2008)*, ed. Agostino Paravicini Bagliani, 55–63. SISMEL – Edizioni del Galluzzo, 2010.

Scholliers, Peter. "Meals, Food Narratives, and Sentiments of Belonging in Past and Present." In *Food, Drink and Identity. Cooking, Eating and Drinking in Europe Since the Middle Ages*, ed. Peter Scholliers, 3–22. Berg, 2001.

Schopen, Armin. *Tinten und Tuschen des arabisch-islamischen Mittelalters. Dokumentation – Analyse – Rekonstruktion*. Vandenhoeck & Ruprecht, 2006.

Schott, Jeremy. "Language." In *Late Ancient Knowing: Explorations in Intellectual History*, ed. Catherine M. Chin and Moulie Vidas, 58–79. University of California Press, 2015.

Schulz, Katja. "Inscriptions in Old Norse Literature." In *Writing Beyond Pen and Parchment. Inscribed Objects in Medieval European Literature*, ed. Ricarda Wagner, Christine Neufeld, and Ludger Lieb, 41–62. De Gruyter, 2019.

Sebo, Erin. "*In scirpo nodum*: Symphosius' Reworking of the Riddle Form." In *The Muse at Play: Riddles and Wordplay in Greek and Latin Poetry*, ed. Jan Kwapzt, David Petrain, and Mikolaj Szymanski, 184–95. De Gruyter, 2013.

Shanzer, Danuta. "Food of Judgement: Late Antiquity and the Early Middle Ages." In *Early Christian Mystagogy and the Body*, ed. Nienke Vos and Paul van Geest, 467–98. Peeters, 2022.

Shapiro, Arthur K., and Elaine Shapiro. *The Powerful Placebo. From Ancient Priest to Modern Physician*. The Johns Hopkins University Press, 1997.

Sharpe, Richard. *Medieval Irish Saints' Lives. An Introduction to Vitae Sanctorum Hiberniae*. Clarendon, 1991.

Sharpe, Richard. "Some Problems Concerning the Organization of the Church in Early Medieval Ireland." *Peritia* 3 (1984): 58–72.

Shaw, Francis. "Medieval Medico-philosophical Treatises in the Irish Language." In *Féil-sgríbhinn Eóin Mhic Néill: Essays and Studies Presented to Professor Eoin MacNeill, D. Litt., on the Occasion of His Seventieth Birthday, May 15th 1938*, ed. John Ryan, 144–57. Three Candles, 1940.

Shupak, Nili. "'Eat This Scroll' (Ezekiel 3:1): Writing as Symbol and Metaphor in the Hebrew Bible in the Light of Ancient Near Eastern Sources." *Bibliotheca Orientalis* 70, no. 1–2 (2013): 25–41.

Simón, Francisco Marco. "Materiality, Oral Incantations and Supernatural Agency in Ancient Healing Magic." *Acta Classica Universitatis Scientiarum Debreceniensis* 57 (2021): 15–42.

Singletary, Keith. "Bay Leaf: Potential Health Benefits." *Nutrition Today* 56, no. 4 (2021): 202–8.

Skemer, Don C. *Binding Words. Textual Amulets in the Middle Ages*. The Pennsylvania State University Press, 2006.

Skemer, Don C. "Magic Writ: Textual Amulets Worn on the Body for Protection." In *Schriftträger – Textträger: Zur materialen Präsenz des Geschriebenen in frühen Gesellschaften*, ed. Annette Kehnel and Diamantis Panagiotopoulos, 127–50. De Gruyter, 2015.

Smith, Mark S. "Evil in Genesis and Other Ancient Near Eastern Creation Stories." In *Narrating the Beginnings*, ed. Alberto Bernabé Pajares and Raquel Martín Hernández, 95–116. Springer, 2021.

Sobott, Robert, Nadine Quenouille, Reinhold Scholl, Klaus Bente, and Christoph Berthold. "Non-Destructive Studies on Ostraca Texts, Inks and Their Ceramic Substrates." In *Archäometrie und Denkmalpflege 2015: Jahrestagung an der Johannes Gutenberg-Universität Mainz, Metalla Sonderheft 7*, ed. T. Gluhak, S. Greiff, K. Kraus and M. Prange, 248–50. Deutsches Bergbau-Museum, 2015.

Sørensen, Jesper. *A Cognitive Theory of Magic*. Altamira Press, 2007.

Sørensen, John Kousgård. "Lægebøger." *Kulturhistorisk leksikon for nordisk middelalder* 2:2 (1982): 76–79.

Spurkland, Terje. "Literacy and 'runacy' in medieval Scandinavia." In *Scandinavia and Europe 800–1350: Contact, Conflict, and Coexistence*, ed. Jonathan Adams and Katherine Holman, 333–44. Brepols, 2004.

Spurkland, Terje. *Norwegian Runes and Runic Inscriptions*, trans. Betsy van der Hoek. The Boydell Press, 2005.

Stephens, John. "The Mead of Poetry." *Neophilologus* 56, no. 3 (1972): 259–68.

Stevens Jr., Phillips. *Rethinking the Anthropology of Magic and Witchcraft. Inherently Human*. Routledge, 2024.

Storms, Godfrid. *Anglo-Saxon Magic*. Springer, 1948 [repr. 2013].

Stuart, Anthony J. "Insularity and Quaternary Vertebrate Faunas in Britain and Ireland." In *Island Britain: A Quaternary Perspective*, ed. Richard C. Preece, 111–25. Geological Society of London, 1995.

Sumler, Alan. "Ingesting Magic: Ingredients and Ecstatic Outcomes in the *Greek* and *Demotic Magical Papyri*." *Arion: A Journal of Humanities and the Classics* 25, no. 1 (2017): 99–126.

Swartz, Michael D. "Magical Piety in Ancient and Medieval Judaism." In *Ancient Magic and Ritual Power*, ed. Marvin Meyer and Paul Mirecki, 167–84. Brill, 2001.

Tambiah, Stanley J. "A Performative Approach to Ritual." *Proceedings of the British Academy* 65 (1979): 113–69.

Tambiah, Stanley J. *Culture, Thought and Social Action*. Harvard University Press, 1985.

Tambiah, Stanley J. "Form and meaning of magical acts. A point of view." *Hau: Journal of Ethnographic Theory* 7, no. 3 (2017): 451–73 (orig. pub. in *Modes of thought: Essays on thinking in Western and non-Western societies*, ed. Robin Horton and Ruth Finnegan [London: Faber & Faber, 1973], 199–229).

Tambiah, Stanley J. *Magic, Science, Religion, and the Scope of Rationality*. Cambridge University Press, 1991.

Tambiah, Stanley J. "The Magical Power of Words." *Man* 3, no. 2 (1968): 175–208.

Tarantola, Arnaud. "Four Thousand Years of Concepts Relating to Rabies in Animals and Humans, Its Prevention and Its Cure." *Tropical Medicine and Infectious Disease* 2, no. 2, 5 (2017), doi: 10.3390/tropicalmed2020005.

Tatomir, Renata-Gabriela. "To Cause 'To Make Divine' Through Smoke: Ancient Egyptian Incense and Perfume. An Inter- and Transdisciplinary Re-Evaluation of Aromatic Biotic Materials Used by the Ancient Egyptians." In *Moesica et Christiana – Studies in honor of Professor Alexandru Barnea*, ed. Adriana Panaite, Romeo Cîrjan, and Carol Căpiţă, 665–78. Muzeul Brăilei "Carol I", Editura Istros, 2016.

ter Horst, Tom. *Codeswitching in the Irish-Latin* Leabhar Breac: *Mediæval Homiletic Culture*. Lot, 2017.

Théodoridès, Jean. "Rabies in Byzantine Medicine." *Dumbarton Oaks Papers, 1984, Vol. 38, Symposium on Byzantine Medicine*, 149–58. Dumbarton Oaks, 1984.

Thorndike, Lynn. "Some Medieval Conceptions of Magic." *The Monist* 25, no. 1 (1915): 107–139.

Thwaite, Annie. "What Is a 'Witch-Bottle'? Assembling the Textual Evidence from Early Modern England." *Magic, Ritual, and Witchcraft* 15, no. 2 (2020): 227–51.

Tolley, Clive. *Shamanism in Norse Myth and Magic*. 2 vols. Academia Scientiarum Fennica, 2009.

Tomczyszyn, Karolina. "'Anoint Your Chest and Eat Some of the Wax-Salve:' The Non-Liturgical Use of Holy Oils in the Early Byzantine East." *Greek, Roman, and Byzantine Studies* 63 (2023): 325–49.

Torfi H. Tulinius. "Egils saga and the novel." In *Snorri Sturluson and the Roots of Nordic Literature: Papers of the International Conference held at "St. Kliment Ohridski" University of Sofia (October 14–16, 2002)*, 117–28. University of Sofia, 2002.

Torfi H. Tulinius. "The Construction of Egil's Saga." In *Egil, the Viking Poet: New Approaches to 'Egils saga'*, ed. Laurence de Looze, Jón Karl Helgason, Russell Poole, and Torfi H. Tulinius, 23–39. University of Toronto Press, 2015.

Torfi H. Tulinius. *The Enigma of Egill. The Saga, the Viking poet, and Snorri Sturluson*, trans. Victoria Cribb. Cornell University Library, 2014.

Torfi H. Tulinius. *The Matter of the North. The Rise of Literary Fiction in Thirteenth-Century Iceland*, trans. Randi C. Eldevik. Odense University Press, 2002.

Totelin, Laurence B. *Taste and the Ancient Senses*. Routledge, 2017.

Trachtenberg, Joshua. *Jewish Magic and Superstition: A Study in Folk Religion*. The University of Pennsylvania Press, 1939.

Tristram, Hildegard L.C. "Feis und fled: Wirklichkeit und Darstellung in mittelalterlichen irischen Gastmahlserzählungen." In *Medialität und mittelalterliche insulare Literatur*, ed. Hildegard L.C. Tristram, 183–220. Narr, 1992.

Tsakos, Alexandros. "Materiality and Physicality of Medieval Manuscripts from Christian Nubia." *Cahiers d'études africaines* 236 (2019): 967–92.

Tzigkounakis, Giorgos, Katerina Simati, and Konstantinos Georgiadis. "The Placebo Effect in Medicine and Clinical Practice: A Narrative Review." *Cureus* Sep 9, 17, 9 (2025): e91893, doi: 10.7759/cureus.91893.

Valente, Luisa. "*Verbum mentis – Vox clamantis*: The Notion of the Mental Word in Twelfth-Century Theology." In *The Word in Medieval Logic, Theology and Psychology. Acts of the XIII International Colloquium of the Société Internationale pour l'étude de la Philosophie Médiévale, Kyoto, 27 September-1 October 2005*, 365–402. Brepols, 2009.

Van Arsdall, Anne. "Medical Training in Anglo-Saxon England." In *Form and Content of Instruction in Anglo-Saxon England in the Light of Contemporary Manuscript Evidence: Papers Presented at the International Conference*, Udine, 6–8 April 2006, ed. Patrizia Lendinara, Loredana Lazzari, and Maria Amalia D'Aronco, 415–35. Brepols, 2007.

Van Arsdall, Anne. "The Transmission of Knowledge in Early Medieval Medical Texts: An Exploration." In *Between Text and Patient: The Medical Enterprise in Medieval and Early Modern Europe*, ed. Florence Eliza Glaze and Brian K. Nance, 201–15. SISMEL – Edizioni del Galluzzo, 2011.

Van Dam, Raymond. *Saints and Their Miracles in Late Antique Gaul*. Princeton University Press, 1993.

van Hamel, Anton Gerard. "The Celtic Grail." *Revue Celtique* 47 (1930): 340–82.

van Liere, Frans. "Biblical Exegesis." In *Handbook of Medieval Studies. Terms – Methods – Trends*, ed. Albert Classen, 5 vols., vol. 1, 137–45. de Gruyter, 2010.

Vassiliev, Afanasiĭ. *Anecdota Graeco-Byzantina*. Universitatis Caesareae, 1893.

Versnel, Henk. "The Poetics of the Magical Charm: An Essay in the Power of Words." In *Magic and Ritual in the Ancient World*, ed. Paul Mirecki and Marvin Meyer, 105–56. Brill, 2002.

Vikan, Gary. "Ruminations on Edible Icons: Originals and Copies in the Art of Byzantium." *Studies in the History of Art* 20 (1989): 47–59.

Vinogradov, Andrey Yu, and Mikhail S. Zheltov. "The 'Apocryphal' Inscription from Mangup, Crimea, and Rituals of 'Exposing the Thief:' Magic and Law from Antiquity to the Middle Ages." *Slověne* 1 (2015): 53–93.

Vitolo, Giovanni. "La Scuola medica salernitana come metafora della storia del Mezzogiorno." *Studi Storici* 45, no. 3 (2004): 633–50.

Voigts, Linda E. "Anglo-Saxon Plant Remedies and the Anglo-Saxons." *Isis* 70 (1979): 250–68.

Voigts, Linda E. "The Character of the Carecter: Ambiguous Sigils in Scientific and Medical Texts." In *Latin and Vernacular: Studies in Late-Medieval Texts and Manuscripts*, ed. Alastair J. Minnis, 91–109. D.S. Brewer, 1989.

von Steinmeyer, Elias, ed. *Die kleineren althochdeutschen Sprachdenkmäler*. Weidmann, 1916.

Waines, David. "Dietetics in Medieval Islamic Culture." *Medical History* 43 (1999): 228–40.

Walker, Harry. "On Logophagy and Truth: Interpretation Through Incorporation among Peruvian Urarina." *Language & Communication* 63 (2018): 15–22.

Walker-Meikle, Kathleen. "Toxicology and Treatment: Medical Authorities and Snake-Bite in the Middle Ages." *Korot -The Israel Journal of the History of Medicine and Science* 22 (2014): 85–104.

Wallis, Faith. "The Experience of the Book: Manuscripts, Texts, and the Role of Epistemology in Early Medieval Medicine." In *Knowledge and the Scholarly Medical Traditions*, ed. Don G. Bates, 101–26. Cambridge University Press, 1995.

Wallis, Faith, ed. *Medieval Medicine. A Reader*. University of Toronto Press, 2010.

Wallis, Faith. "Gregory of Tours' Nosebleed." In *Une traversée des savoirs. Mélanges offerts à Jackie Pigeaud*, ed. Philippe Heuzé, Yves Herant, and Éric Van Der Schueren, 417–36. Presses de l'Université Laval, 2008.

Wallis, Robert J. "Witchcraft and Magic in the Age of Anthropology." In *The Oxford Illustrated History of Witchcraft and Magic*, ed. Owen Davies, 225–52. Oxford University Press, 2017.

Wanner, Kevin. *Snorri Sturluson and the Edda. The Conversion of Cultural Capital in Medieval Scandinavia*. University of Toronto Press, 2008.

Ware III, Rudolph T. *The Walking Qur'an: Islamic Education, Embodied Knowledge, and History in West Africa*. The University of North Carolina Press, 2014.

Warren, Meredith J.C. "Tasting the Little Scroll: A Sensory Analysis of Divine Interaction in Revelation 10.8–10." *Journal for the Study of the New Testament* 40, no. 1 (2017): 101–19.

Wasik, Bill, and Monica Murphy. *Rabid. A Cultural History of the World's Most Diabolical Virus*. Viking, 2012.

Watkins, Carl. "'Folklore' and 'Popular Religion' in Britain during the Middle Ages." *Folklore* 115, no. 2 (2004): 140–50.

Wehlau, Ruth. "Rumination and Re-Creation: Poetic Instruction in *The Order of the World*." *Florilegium* 13 (1994): 65–77.

Weill-Parot, Nicolas. "Imprinting Powers: The Astrological Seal and Its Doctrinal Meanings in the Latin West." *The Medieval Globe* 4, no. 1 (2018): 49–72.

West, Philip J. "Rumination in Bede's Account of Cædmon." *Monastic Studies* 12 (1976): 217–26.

Wilson, Stephen. "Introduction." In Id., *Saints and their Cults. Studies in Religious Sociology, Folklore and History*, 1–54. Cambridge University Press, 1983.

Wiśniewski, Robert. *The Beginnings of the Cult of Relics*. Oxford University Press, 2019.

Wöhrle, Georg. "Papyrophagie." In *"… vor dem Papyrus sind alle gleich!". Papyrologische Beiträge zu Ehren von Bärbel Kramer (P. Kramer)*, ed. Eberhard Raimar, Holger Kockelman, Stefan Pfeiffer, and Maren Schentuleit, 243–47. de Gruyter, 2009.

Wood, Ian. "The problem of late Merovingian culture." In *Exzerpieren – Kompilieren – Tradieren: Transformationen des Wissens zwischen Spätantike und Frühmittelalter*, ed. Stephan Dusil, Gerald Schwedler, and Raphael Schwitter, 199–222. De Gruyter, 2017.

Wormald, Patrick. *Papers Preparatory to the Making of English Law: King Alfred to the Twelfth Century*, vol. 2. University of London, 2014.

Wycherley, Niamh. *The Cult of Relics in Early Medieval Ireland*, Studies in the Early Middle Ages 43. Brepols, 2015.

Xhayet, Geneviève. *Médecine et arts divinatoires dans le monde bénédictin médiéval d'après les réceptaires de Saint-Jacques de Liège*. Garnier, 2010.

Yelle, Robert A. "Rhetorics of Law and Ritual: A Semiotic Comparison of the Law of Talion and Sympathetic Magic." *Journal of the American Academy of Religion* 69, no. 3 (2001): 627–48.

Yuhong, Wu. "Rabies and Rabid Dogs in Sumerian and Akkadian Literature." *Journal of the American Oriental Society* 121, no. 1 (2001): 32–43.

Zadeh, Travis. "Touching and Ingesting: Early Debates over the Material Qur'an." *Journal of the American Oriental Society* 129, no. 3 (2009): 446–66.

Zaffagno, Elena. "Il giuramento scritto sulla mela." *Materiali e contributi per la storia della narrativa greca* 1 (1976): 109–19.

Zusne, Leonard, and Warren H. Jones. *Anomalistic Psychology: A Study of Magical Thinking*. L. Erlbaum, 1989.

Index of Names

 | HTTPS://DOI.ORG/10.1163/9789004765528-010

Index of Places

 | HTTPS://DOI.ORG/10.1163/9789004765528-011

www.ingramcontent.com/pod-product-compliance
Lightning Source LLC
Chambersburg PA
CBHW071339230926
51846CB00002B/388
9789004765498